# THE
# CRYSTAL
## CODE

# THE
# CRYSTAL
## CODE

## TAMARA DRIESSEN

PENGUIN LIFE

AN IMPRINT OF

PENGUIN BOOKS

PENGUIN LIFE

UK | USA | Canada | Ireland | Australia
India | New Zealand | South Africa

Penguin Life is part of the Penguin Random House
group of companies whose addresses can be found at
global.penguinrandomhouse.com.

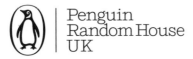

First published 2018
001

Copyright © Tamara Driessen, 2018

Photography by Kristina Sälgvik

The moral right of the copyright holders has been asserted

Designed and typeset by Hampton Associates
Colour reproduction by Rhapsody
Printed in China

A CIP catalogue record for this book is available from the British Library

ISBN: 978-0-241-34697-6

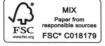

MIX
Paper from
responsible sources
FSC® C018179

Penguin Random House is committed to a sustainable
future for our business, our readers and our planet. This book
is made from Forest Stewardship Council® certified paper.

# CONTENTS

# INTRODUCTION

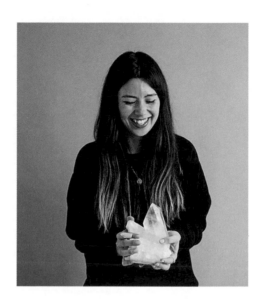

Crystals have a way of magnetizing us, and it can happen in the most random places. Once, I was boarding a plane with my boyfriend – we were on our way home after four days of exploring Ibiza. We'd queued for what felt like for ever to board, and now we were waiting to find our seats on that no-frills aircraft. As a man reached up to put his bag in the overhead locker, my gaze was drawn to the huge Fluorite pendant he was wearing. I couldn't take my eyes off it. 'I love your crystal!' I said. I was *trying* to play it cool and suppress my inner Gollum. He just nodded. I slunk into my seat.

I can't help it. A crystal gets me every time. My eyes just want to be on it. I know I'm not the only person this happens to. There's always a sense of familiarity, like being reunited with a long-lost friend – 'Where have you been all this time?'

Perhaps a few crystals have found their way into your life and their magnetic pull makes you want to keep them close. They may feel as if they fit perfectly with you and your life as you hold them; the missing piece to your jigsaw puzzle.

The thing is, they're more than just lucky rocks.

I must have been about eight when I bought my first crystal. We were on a half-term trip to the Natural History Museum in London. I chose a light pink Rose Quartz instead of a dinosaur stationery set from the gift shop. I loved that rock because, although I didn't know why, it comforted me. Since then, I've always had at least one crystal at my side – or in my bra.

As a teenager I'd carry a piece of Tiger's Eye so that I'd feel more confident – it gave me the courage to ignore the bullies in my class. And I bought myself a Garnet ring from Elizabeth Duke in the Argos catalogue because I'd read in one of my nineties teen magazines that it would attract a boyfriend. It worked!

In my twenties, I had a constant knot of anxiety that I'd attempt to numb with food, partying and being a chronic people-pleaser. I felt as if I was constantly chasing my tail, trying to escape my inner critic. I thought that if I made everyone else happy, I'd be happy. I was wrong. Amethyst and Citrine were my allies in overcoming regular panic attacks, anxiety, depression and a long-term eating disorder. These crystals have calmed my overactive mind, decluttered my thoughts and guided me to trusting that I deserve to be happy before anything else.

While my collection has grown, I've learnt more about crystals through my personal practice, and from the crystals I've intuitively given to friends, with notes of their powers – always confirmed to be the medicine they needed.

A few years ago Lee, one of my housemates, was holding my beloved Clear Quartz cluster: 'How do they make them? Are they stuck together?'

No one had ever asked me this before. 'They're mostly formed when the earth began, and some take millions of years to form, in caves or underground.' I googled the Selenite Cave in Mexico to show him what I meant. It can be hard to believe that these formations are native to our own planet when you think of the urban jungles a lot of us live in.

He zoomed into the picture for a better look. 'Why doesn't yours look like this cave?'

'Crystals are made of minerals, and every crystal has its own composition, which gives it its colour and shape. This also depends on where in the world they form. Like, different countries or places have different terrains. Some are man-made but the natural ones are my favourites.' I showed him a piece of rainbow-infused crystal – Angel Aura – so that he could compare the difference between a heat-treated crystal and a natural specimen.

'But why do you have so many? What do you do with them?'

'I use them for healing. They're full of good vibes.'

He wasn't convinced.

'According to scientists, they're made of particles that hold energy. These particles are tightly compacted but have the smallest amount of space for movement, which can emit a vibration. Even though we can't see it, crystals vibrate.' I knew he suffered from anxiety and offered to make him a crystal healing elixir – water infused with the energy of crystals. He was open to the idea and drank it to humour me. The next day he asked me to make it for him again, and 'borrowed' some of my crystals.

My affinity with the realm of crystals has led me to study various crystal bibles and guides, attend crystal healing workshops and courses, and explore the power of crystals with a shaman in Bali. I wanted to consolidate what I was learning with facts and confirmed knowledge so that I could work with crystals as a professional healer and share what I was discovering.

Every crystal has its own personality that can initially be interpreted through colour, shape, the amount of light that shines through it or, if it's opaque, how much light it absorbs. (See the Crystal Guide, page 111). Likewise, I believe that the crystals you choose say a lot about *your* personality and pursuits.

Although I have a vast selection of crystals, I'm drawn to some again and again. It's like when you buy a new lipstick: you feel amazing when you try it on but when you get home you realize it's more or less the same as all the others in your make-up bag. I went through a stage of doing this with Amethyst. I'm an Aries and a born over-thinker. During my teens and twenties I overanalysed everything – the way I looked, the things I said, the decisions I made, how I perceived the way other people acted towards me. It was exhausting. I was blocked from my intuition because my brain was so cluttered. That was until Amethyst came along. Whenever I connect with Amethyst, everything slows down and time seems to expand. The words 'Chill out' come to mind.

I believe that when you're drawn to a crystal on repeat, it's a sign that this is what you need. It's guiding you towards something exciting! Which crystals are predominant in your collection? What are they showing you? It's time to take action!

Crystals can be seen as the physical embodiment of your intentions. We choose them because they promise us something that resonates with our current situation and aspirations. You could choose Peacock Ore to invoke more confidence for a Tinder date, Citrine to cheer you on as you pluck up the courage to ask for the pay rise you've been waiting for, Black Tourmaline to protect you from draining work politics, Celestite to calm your anxiety, Moonstone to soothe PMT, Kunzite to get over your ex and Rose Quartz to hold your hand as you nurture a more loving relationship with yourself. If there's a feeling you want to experience, there's a crystal to encourage it.

Before I met my boyfriend, I slept next to a selection of crystals – let's call it a love spell. I'd taken a break from the dating scene so that I could focus on learning to love myself – instigated by a series of disastrous relationships. During the break, I created a clear intention of the kind of relationship I wanted to be in, how I wanted to feel with him, and chose crystals that reflected what I was aiming for.

I chose two pieces of Rose Quartz (to represent the two of us), Pink Kunzite because it's said to help you find new love after a break-up, Garnet for commitment and Clear Quartz to remove any blocks. I programmed the crystals with my intention and slept with them next to me so that I could energetically align myself with the frequency of what I was calling in. Six weeks later, I met the love of my life. We live together now and I've had to cut down on the number of crystals I sleep with, mainly because they find their way to his side of the bed and wake him up in the night.

These days I sleep with Moonstone and Lepidolite on my bedside table to help me keep dreaming through the night and align me to my energetic cycles so that life can flow as it needs to.

Every crystal has its own superpowers, but if you try to work with too many at once, it's like being overloaded with advice by a gang of well-meaning friends. As everyone has their own spin on things, you're overwhelmed and don't know where to start.

Your healing journey needs to happen one day at a time. With crystals, you'll get the most out of them when you commit to working with one or a few at a time. You need the one that feels magnetized to you. Forget the dusty description. Instead listen to the one that calls to you the loudest, regardless of any logical reason.

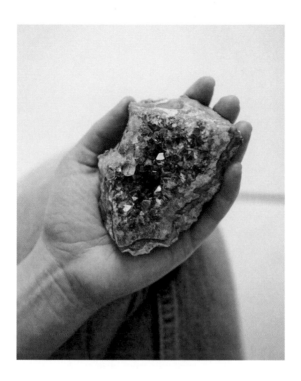

Close your eyes and hold a crystal in your non-dominant hand. How does it feel? Do you notice any shifts in your energy? Tune into the crystal that you're drawn to today. The one that you don't want to let go. That's the one for you.

The crystals you're drawn to can change every day because you naturally feel different each day – or even hour. Some days you'll feel inspired, sociable and creative. On others you'll feel introverted, tired and passive. That's the ebb and flow of life. It's normal to feel like that. Choosing one crystal will help you feel more centred.

I've seen the subtle shifts that have occurred in my life from the presence of crystals and realized that they're a catalyst for bigger transformation. I'm always learning more from these unassuming 'rocks' and am constantly in awe of the chain of events that follows from connecting with them. Now I run my own crystal-healing practice and lead crystal-healing workshops because I love sharing this journey with others.

Recently, I held a Full Moon Ceremony using Smoky Quartz, which is known for protection and grounding. It's also known for pain relief. I know that sounds totally woo-woo – how can a crystal do ibuprofen's job? I didn't believe it myself until that day.

I'd had a cold but I felt well enough to lead the ceremony. My throat still felt uncomfortable and I was drinking a lot of hot water with lemon, manuka honey and ginger (which wasn't making much difference). I meditated with Smoky Quartz in the morning to prepare for the evening ahead, and when I sat up I discovered that my throat felt better. Surely it was just coincidence? One of the regulars to the ceremony suffers from fibromyalgia and wanted to get to know Smoky Quartz for pain relief. I knew what had happened to me and hoped it could work for her.

A week later Rebecca tagged me in a post on Instagram:

> I have felt particularly connected to Smoky Quartz, strong visualizations in the meditation and messages from the oracle spread. Also, it's said that Smoky Quartz relieves pain. I've slept with the crystal in my hand for four out of the last seven nights and the reduction in my pain has been crazy. I'm currently feeling the best I've felt since August last year. Normally on a day like today, where it's raining, I'd be in so much pain and struggling at work, but I managed to sit at my desk all day with minimal pain! There's a sceptical part of my brain shouting, 'It's just good timing,' but there's another part whispering, 'What if . . .?'

This is why I've been inspired to work consistently with one or a few crystals at a time so that I get the most from them. When you focus on a chosen few, the shifts are more apparent because the practice is more concentrated. When you cleanse them regularly, meditate and keep them close by, you get to know the crystals in your hand. You start seeing life through them. A crystal's support is unconditional, and all of them work much more efficiently when we give them some TLC – leaving them to roll around in the bottom of your handbag isn't enough. That's when a crystal becomes an ornament, its power lying dormant.

Crystal healing isn't a new concept. Some ancient civilizations are believed to have been built around the power of crystals – like Atlantis. Lapis Lazuli is associated with the Egyptian sky goddess, Isis, and Cleopatra was said to wear crushed Lapis Lazuli as eyeshadow to promote spiritual consciousness. To the Ancient Greeks *amethystos* was a stone of sobriety, used to prevent drunkenness and addictions. Vedic astrologers have historically prescribed gemstones to empower weak planetary alignments and strengthen the physical body.

So, this is a call to action. Don't leave your crystals to get dusty. It's time to work with them and find out what the hype's about. Crystals unlock the power within you, a power that was there all along. The kind of power where you become your own muse. When you work on yourself, and surrender to the process, you become the person you've been waiting to be. You stop needing external validation and start doing things because you want to.

In this book you'll find a guide to seventy crystals. Each has a description that includes what it's commonly known for. The messages are intuitively interpreted from my connection to the crystal with the intention to guide and empower you. You'll learn how to work with your crystals through simple rituals and initiations so that you can experience the benefits of crystal healing. This book is intended as a catalyst for you to cultivate a relationship with yourself through crystals and beyond, inviting more mindfulness into your life to support you in tuning into what you need. Some crystals and practices may inspire you more than others. There will be crystals that just aren't for you – and others that may surprise you. If you don't have the specified crystals or other items, feel free to improvise and be creative, rather than not doing the rituals/practice/meditation.

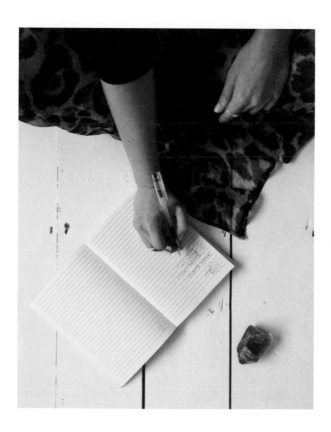

# PORTABLE MAGIC

**This book can be used as an oracle, through the ancient process of bibliomancy (divination through books). All the crystals you need are waiting for you between these pages. Sit somewhere quiet where you won't be disturbed, close your eyes and take a few calming breaths, allowing your thoughts to slow. Tune mindfully into the moment of now. Hold the book close to you and, when you feel ready, choose a page at random to select a crystal to guide you. Read the page you've intuitively selected and be open to how the crystal's message represents itself to you throughout the day.**

I'd recommend keeping a crystal journal and be liberal with your notes. Write about what inspires you from working with crystals and the shifts you notice – otherwise you're likely to forget, and nothing beats reading notes to your future self.

Maybe you've picked up this book because you're looking for your big break from the universe – you're ready to check out of Heartbreak Hotel, there's no room for anxiety any more and you're bored with comparing your life to everyone else's picture-perfect Instagram showreels. Right now a one-way ticket to Bali isn't an option so you may as well find out what the crystals are saying. Welcome! Working with crystals is an invitation to step into your own power. This is about you . . . and your crystal ally, in whatever form it may be.

Some say that crystals are magic. I believe they're more than that. They have the power to reveal your truest self, the version of you that's been waiting to be acknowledged. It's time to blow away the cobwebs and get to know your crystals.

# CHAPTER ONE

# CRYSTALS 101

## WHAT ARE CRYSTALS?

You may be wondering! Some look like unassuming rocks (see Orange Calcite, page 145), others as if they're from outer space (see Aragonite, page 129), and many are almost guaranteed to make you swoon for the way light shines through them (see Optical Calcite, page 142) or the flashes of ethereal colours you see as you move them around (see Labradorite, page 189). A crystal is defined by specific characteristics, but the word 'crystal' is often used interchangeably with 'rock', 'gemstone' and 'stone'. All crystals have one thing in common: they're formed from minerals through varying processes, which account for the differences between them. Real crystals are distinguished from the rest of the natural world by their unique internal geometric structure. You could think of crystals as the flowers of the mineral world, because of their beauty. Healers work with rocks, gemstones, stones, crystals and other natural elements because they're all valuable for their transformative superpowers.

## MINERALS

A mineral is defined as solid matter with a specific chemical composition, made directly by Mother Earth and inorganic – which means that it contains no trace of anything that was once living, like fossilized plants or animals. Minerals have an internal crystalline structure – although this can't always be seen by the naked eye – which means that their molecules are arranged in an orderly geometric pattern.

**Examples of minerals**: Kyanite, Lepidolite, Fuchsite, Malachite

## CRYSTALS

'Legit' crystals are easily recognized by their eye-catching formations. Most have naturally smooth facets, points and angles, like Amethyst and Celestite. High-quality crystals will have a glass-like clarity. All of the quartz family are crystals, even Rose Quartz, which is usually found in chunks. Pyrite is also known as a crystal because of its unique geometric formations. Here's the science: when you look at a crystal, you're seeing the result of molecular patterns that are aligned geometrically to create a three dimensional cohesive and symmetric or asymmetric form. These formations can be mesmerizing and their beauty is treasured universally – some people are surprised that Mother Earth forms them!

**Examples of crystals**: Quartz, Apophyllite, Celestite, Pyrite

## ROCKS

Rocks are a mixture of different minerals fused together to form a solid mass. They're usually a combination of several minerals but can contain just one, which is less common. You can usually tell: if a rock has more than one colour it's composed of more than one mineral. Lapis Lazuli is a great example: the blue is Lazurite; if it has white in it, that's often Calcite, and any gold flecks are Pyrite. Rocks are different from minerals because they may contain the remnants of living things, like Septarian.

**Examples of rocks**: Septarian, Lapis Lazuli, Unakite, Obsidian

## GEMSTONES

Gemstones are precious or semi-precious stones, prized for their rarity and clarity. Many are strong enough to be mechanically enhanced: they are are cut and faceted, using grinding and polishing techniques to create specific angles and shapes. These processes enhance how the light travels through a stone to maximize its radiance so that it can be used in jewellery and other forms of adornment. Take a trip to the Tower of London to see the Crown Jewels, one of the world's most famous gemstone collections.

**Examples of gemstones**: Diamond, Emerald, Amethyst, Moonstone

# WHERE DO CRYSTALS COME FROM?

**The life of a crystal begins deep within the earth, conceived through heat and pressure. Below the earth's surface, tectonic plates float between its crust and the mantle below it – it's so hot down there that the temperature can reach 900°C.**

As the tectonic plates crash together, they cause stress fractures, folds and faults, which can result in earthquakes and the creation of mountains. It also encourages molten rock to rise closer to the earth's surface, where the minerals cool and crystallize as they solidify.

Have you heard of Crystal Castle and Shambhala Gardens in Australia? It's Disneyland for crystal junkies. Imagine lush subtropical gardens filled with towering crystals, statues, labyrinths, fossils and the world's largest Amethyst cave. The 'Enchanted Cave' is the result of a giant bubble that formed inside molten lava, 120 million years ago. The extreme heat and pressure combined with iron to create millions of tiny Amethyst crystals, which cover the internal walls of the bubble. It was discovered by a farmer in Uruguay, South America, before it was brought to Crystal Castle. The best part? You can sit and meditate inside the Enchanted Cave! A trip to Australia may seem out of reach, but I'd recommend an internet search for 'Crystal Castle and Shambhala Gardens: Enchanted Cave' so that you can see how crystals are formed.

As each crystal journeys to you, it absorbs nature's elements: air, water, fire and earth. Its personality is determined by where it formed, its chemical composition, structure and the process it went through. So, crystals associated with fire will inspire action and passion; water will encourage you to access your subconscious and intuition; air will bring clarity and enhance communication; earth will guide you to feel more grounded and supported in the present moment. These elements are medicine from Mother Earth and we need a balance of them in our own lives. Each crystal encapsulates the healing energies she offers us – a portable dose of medicine that you can take wherever you go. There are times when you're 'too busy' to go outside for some headspace and walk barefoot on the grass or among trees. You could think of crystals as a lazy person's way of connecting with the elements.

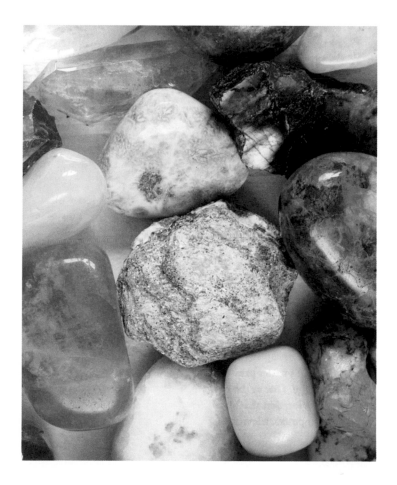

Synthetic crystals and minerals are created in laboratories, and while some are beautiful, they lack the energies that have accumulated in natural crystals through their formation – just as processed food doesn't contain the same nutrients as raw. They're often made for manufacturing purposes, which eliminates any inconsistencies, like inclusions from other materials, to ensure a specific composition. Artificial crystals offer a cheaper alternative to the real thing. For example, synthetic quartz is used in watches.

# HOW DO CRYSTALS WORK?

**Side-glancing sceptics often ask this question! It's important to have the full lowdown on how these beauties work so that we can appreciate all of the wonderful ways that crystals can weave their magic in our lives.**

I understand that crystals having the ability to affect your emotions and give you more confidence may seem crazy to some, but few people question how other seemingly ordinary things work. You may consider some of our most used gadgets to be pretty mysterious and magical. Think of your mobile phone: a portable device that enables you to speak to someone (almost) anywhere in the world. It stores all kinds of information from your holiday photos to your to-do lists. It can improve your mood because it gives you access to laugh-out-loud memes and is programmed with apps to support your everyday life. Unless the phone is plugged in to charge, it doesn't require any visible wires or connections to do its thing. Would you be surprised if I told you that this couldn't happen without crystals?

Electronic devices are made with minerals, like copper, gold, silver and platinum, alongside quartz crystal that's programmed as silicon chips to process the information we type on a keyboard or tap on a screen. Quartz crystal can create piezoelectricity. This means that when it's under pressure, through heat, movement or impact, it releases a gentle electrical charge. Due to the crystal's geometric structure, the electrical charge creates an oscillating vibration that's stable, accurate and consistent. It's used in other modern tools, like computers, televisions, radios, medical equipment, lasers, watches and satellites.

Other crystals, like Ruby, are used in lasers because they produce a 'coherent visible light'. Ruby itself supports us with laser-like focus and commitment to our passion projects. Tourmaline is used in hair straighteners because it emits negative ions that neutralize the positive ions in dry or damaged hair to make it easier to style with less heat. In a similar way it's known to ground and protect our energy, thus making our lives, not just our hair, easier to manage. Fluorite is used to produce hydrofluoric acid, which the steel industry harnesses to remove impurities and to fuse metals together. It's also incorporated in the non-stick coating on cooking pans, which is interesting: it's associated with psychic self-defence and purifying the aura.

Crystals play a vital role in our technological revolution because they focus, store, transmit and transform energy. You could say that we're living in the Crystal Age. With this in mind, is it so out-there to believe that crystals have the power to support us emotionally, spiritually and physically?

Albert Einstein famously said, 'Everything in life is a vibration.' Yes, that means you, me and everything around us. What we perceive as our physical and material world is composed of particles vibrating at different frequencies. These frequencies, a.k.a. vibrations, influence what we see and hear, and how we feel, because we're constantly interacting with our environment as energy.

# 'Everything in life is a vibration'

## ALBERT EINSTEIN

As humans, our atomic structure and frequency are considered to be unstable because we're always moving, changing, regenerating, healing, ageing, emotionally fluid, experiencing different things. We're in a constant state of transformation. We're also very susceptible, and our energy tunes into the world around us through 'entrainment' in which we synchronize with an external rhythm. You could think of it as tuning into different radio stations, or how your mood changes depending on who you're with or what's happening around you. When you're sitting in the car and all of a sudden your favourite song is playing, your mood lifts in an instant. Compare that with how you feel after interacting with a rude barista (who's just having a bad day, to which everyone is entitled) – you can't help but feel disgruntled as you walk away with your matcha latte. They're both entrainment in action.

# DEFINITION OF
# ENTRAINMENT:

**when a person synchronizes with
an external influence, which affects
how they feel, act and move.**

When a crystal is working its magic, the effects can be subtle. It may take you a little while to notice the benefits if you aren't paying attention. Just as you won't instantly be fluent in Spanish because you've signed up to a course, a crystal won't transform your life because you've bought it and left it on your bedside table. Through the process of entrainment, crystals can recalibrate our energy, due to their stable frequency. Their colour adds another dimension to their personality. When we feel calm and centred, we open up to new experiences and have a deeper sense of awareness. Crystals may be inanimate but they send out vibrations. The key to unlocking their power is to use them consciously and consistently. (See Crystal Rituals, page 63). As with anything rewarding, it takes time and care.

A crystal can act as a talisman and serve as a reminder of something you're consciously aiming for or invoking. Seeing the crystal regularly – on your altar (see page 72), beside your bed, on your desk, in a pendant or ring – and aligning with it can help you stay focused, especially when you think, How can I embody the personality of the crystal in this situation? That can help you stay on track to achieving your goals. Crystals can assist you in becoming the most evolved version of yourself by nudging you to realize your highest potential.

# CRYSTAL HUNTING, A.K.A. HIGH-VIBE RETAIL THERAPY

**How do you choose your crystals? Is it a speed-dating kinda thing where you read all of the micro-descriptions and see what the crystal feels like when you hold it? Or is it love at first sight, as if you've been reunited with your crystalline soulmate?**

There's no right or wrong way to choose crystals. The most important thing is that you feel a connection. You could set an intention before you walk into the shop (and ask your highest self, spirit guides, angels or deities to guide you, if this resonates with you) and ask to be shown a crystal that will support you. It doesn't have to be the prettiest, or the most expensive, to rock your world. Sometimes it's the unlikeliest that provides the boost you need. Give the one that magnetizes you a chance, the one that stops you in your tracks, the one you can't take your eyes off or your hands are drawn to. It's easier said than done but try not to over-think your choice – you can't choose wrong when it comes to crystals.

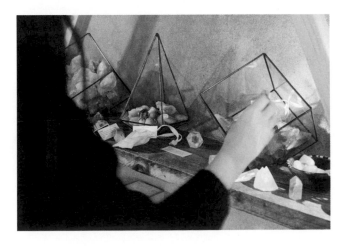

# FIVE SIGNS THAT YOU'VE FOUND YOUR CRYSTAL:

- **Sense of calm/reassurance/clarity/familiarity/ confidence/inner knowing/excitement/grounding**
- **Love at first sight**
- **The Gollum effect –** *my precious*: **you don't want to put it down and seem to be hypnotized because you can't stop looking at it**
- **It may not be the one you thought you were looking for but you're drawn to it no matter how many other crystals you look at**
- **The ultimate sign that you've chosen the 'right' one: it's coming home with you**

## INTERNET CRYSTAL SHOPPING

The world of crystal shopping has opened up with a little help from the internet and an abundance of crystal dealers offering exotic specimens that you may not find in your usual haunts. The same rules apply as when you're choosing a crystal in a shop: you can't hold it before you buy it, but if you're drawn to a particular crystal and keep landing back on its page, it's the one. When you're buying from a website, it's important to keep in mind that you may not receive the exact crystal in the listing. Check the product description to avoid disappointment. Some crystals can look bigger in the picture than they actually are, and sometimes the picture is a show crystal so you will receive one of its brothers or sisters. That being said, there are some wonderful online crystal shops that consistently provide high-quality crystals: what you see is what you get. If in doubt, make sure you ask before you click 'buy now'.

## BUYING CRYSTALS FOR OTHER PEOPLE

Take a few moments before you go into the shop or start browsing the page to visualize your friend next to you and consider how you'd like the crystal to support him or her. You could call on your highest self, spirit guides, angels, deities or your heart to guide you to a crystal for them. Certain crystals are associated with specific situations but be guided by what your intuition is saying.

## WHICH CRYSTALS ARE MOST POWERFUL?

This is totally subjective and the answer is simple: the crystal you're most drawn to and with which you choose to collaborate is the most powerful. Crystals only work when you do. You and your intention give the crystal its true power. Moldavite is highly esteemed as a stone of transformation but I don't get the hype. I've experimented with it in my meditations but it doesn't resonate with me at the moment. Amethyst and Moonstone, though, have inspired huge shifts in my life. There'll be a crystal for a reason, a season and a lifetime: they are all powerful at the perfect time. The crystals I trust to be the most powerful are the ones I've actively collaborated with. There will be crystals that never cross my path but may become big players in your crystal journey. So, any crystal that you're drawn to and that you focus on working with will be the most powerful for *you*.

## DOES SIZE MATTER?

With crystals, bigger does not necessarily equal higher potency. Of course, larger specimens can have a more obvious presence and make a statement, but if a small crystal finds its way to you it can still have the wow factor. It goes without saying that extra-large crystals are definitely less portable, which may restrict how you work with them – you'd risk an injury trying to balance a large cluster on your third eye for a meditation! They'd be more suitable for keeping indoors where they can bring positive vibes to your home, workspace or altar (see page 72). Smaller crystals, like tumbled stones and crystal points, are ideal for travelling, wearing as jewellery, making crystal elixirs (page 96), meditating with (page 64) or doing layouts (page 90).

Remember: size doesn't matter, it's what you do with your crystals that counts.

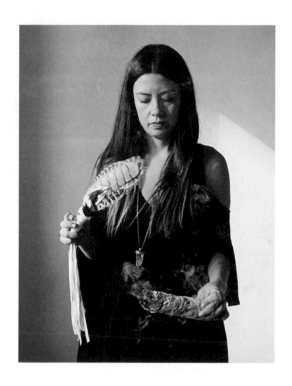

# CRYSTAL MAINTENANCE

## HOW TO ACTIVATE YOUR CRYSTAL

As soon as you buy your crystal, it's important to cleanse your new friend. Crystals absorb and transmute all kinds of energy and it helps them to have a fresh start. I like to think of crystals as cosmic technology, similar to your iPhone: when you update the software and get your apps in order, everything runs to full effect. The same goes for crystals.

Cleansing a crystal is like sending its current data to the universal hard drive: programming it will update the software, and charging gives it the power boost it needs. Until you do this, you're sitting on untapped potential.

## HOW TO CLEANSE YOUR CRYSTALS

### Sacred smoke, a.k.a. smudging

Dried herbs, plants and wood, like white sage, palo santo and sweetgrass are considered sacred plants, according to shamanic traditions and other ancient cultures; they are used for protection, purification and grounding. Recent scientific studies have shown that medicinal smoke can rid the air of harmful bacteria. Burning these herbs also has an uplifting effect: it neutralizes the charge of positive ions by releasing large amounts of negative ions into the space.

An ion is an electrically charged particle formed when its atoms have either lost or gained electrons (lost electron = positive ion; gained electron = negative ion). Even though we can't see them, ions are floating everywhere. The electromagnetic field (aura) around our body and environment can accumulate positive ions, which may have a detrimental effect by causing us to feel overwhelmed, lethargic and burnt out. Positive ions are triggered in nature by strong winds, storms, humidity and pollution, and by fluorescent lights, electrical devices and equipment, home appliances and hairdryers. Negative ions are abundant in nature, in forests and other places where plants are photosynthesizing, and near moving water – this is one of the reasons why connecting with nature can be so restorative for us and why keeping plants in your home can be beneficial, especially when you remember to water them! Living busy lives in urban jungles can restrict our access to these natural highs, and simple tricks, like smudging, can offer a quick fix to bring some balance into our lives (and our crystals).

The smoke from sage or palo santo will neutralize any energy stored by the crystal. It is a quick and easy way to cleanse crystals and ideal for crystals that aren't suited to water, such as Selenite, Pyrite, Opal and Peacock Ore.

Light your sage or palo santo and allow it to burn for a few moments. Once the flame has disappeared, let the smoke flow over the crystal.

### Running water

We all know the benefits of washing in water, and most crystals dig it to wash away any unwanted energy.

Hold your crystal under running water for a few minutes or until it feels refreshed. This could be from a tap in the sink or in a stream (just be careful you don't lose your crystal down the plughole or drop it in the stream). Visualize the water washing away any unwanted energy.

## Salt water

Salt has been used by witches, Ancient Egyptians and in folk magic or Buddhist practices because it absorbs negative energy. It's often used in rituals for purification and protection.

- Fill a bowl with water and add two big pinches of natural salt, preferably pink Himalayan.

- Once the salt has dissolved, immerse the crystal in the water. Leave it for a few hours or overnight, then rinse it with fresh water and allow it to dry.

- If you have crystal set in jewellery that you want to cleanse but are worried about damaging it in salt water, you can use an indirect method: fill the bowl with water (as above) and place a small tumbler in the bowl allowing the water to surround it without overflowing into it. Place your jewellery in the glass where it will remain dry but will absorb the cleansing intention from the surrounding water.

Some crystals can be damaged by contact with water and/or salt – for example, Selenite, Pyrite, Lapis Lazuli, Haematite and Opal. If in doubt, follow the indirect method, smudging, visualization, or rest the crystal on a large quartz cluster to prevent any adverse effects.

## Visualization

There will be times when you want to freshen up your crystal while you have no access to the items suggested. Your intention is actually one of the most powerful tools you have in your 'tool-kit', which means you don't necessarily need a collection of witchy paraphernalia. Instead, you can project your intention by using this simple visualization technique, any time and anywhere you choose.

Hold your crystal and visualize pure white light flowing in through the top of your head, down into your heart, spreading across your chest and through your arms, to your hands and into the crystal. Visualize the pure white light cleansing the crystal and removing any unwanted energy.

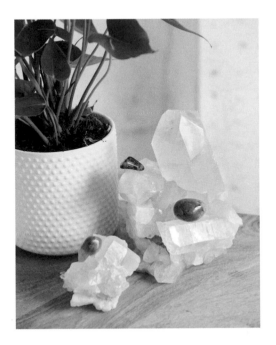

## Large quartz cluster

Quartz clusters big enough to hold other crystals may be used for cleansing because they can absorb and transform energy. To cleanse your everyday crystals or jewellery, leave them on a large cluster overnight: they will be fresh to use the next day. I'd suggest a large Clear Quartz or Citrine cluster for this purpose.

Use one of the cleansing techniques mentioned above to clear the cluster regularly and programme it with the intention to cleanse your crystals and jewellery of any energy that doesn't belong to or serve you.

## Essential oils

Essential oils capture the essence of flowers, herbs and roots; the oil carries the plant's scent. These fragrances act as plant medicine: they can elevate our senses and are stimulating to us and to crystals. I prefer to use organic essential oils so that I know they aren't mixed with anything synthetic that might damage the crystal. When you use essential oils to cleanse your crystals, you'll be giving them a boost from Mother Earth herself.

Either add a few drops of essential oil to water and immerse the crystal, or place a few drops on a clean cloth and gently wipe it. For their cleansing properties, sage, rosemary, sandalwood, frankincense, lavender and palo santo oils are particularly suited to this purpose, but feel free to use your favourite oils.

## Crystal cleansing spray

A range of crystal cleansing sprays is available and they're ideal for freshening your crystals without fuss. Check out page 108 to find out how to make your own.

## Moonbathing

Let your crystals soak up some moonlight. Leave them on a windowsill or in your garden overnight to reset and recharge, during a full moon, if possible, because it's a time that represents abundance, gratitude and celebration. It's thought to be a potent time, and plugging your crystals into the full moon's energy will infuse them with plenty of moon juice.

It doesn't have to be a full moon: crystals love nature so putting them outside to connect with any moon phase that feels good for you will work wonders.

## Self-cleansing crystals

Some popular resources talk about 'self-cleansing' crystals, which suggests that they don't require cleansing and their energy can cleanse other crystals. These include Natural Citrine, Selenite and Kyanite. There doesn't seem to be any scientific evidence to show why these crystals have this ability while others don't but, equally, there isn't much scientific research behind a lot of metaphysical practices. As always, experiment with your crystals and tune into what feels right for you.

## HOW OFTEN DO I NEED TO CLEANSE MY CRYSTALS?

I'd always recommend cleansing a crystal when you first get it, and before you use it for a meditation, ritual or layout. You could think of it in the same way as washing your hands before eating – good-vibe hygiene is just as important. The rest is up to you, how much time you have available and how many crystals you have in your collection. When you notice that your crystals' powers are a bit sluggish or they seem lacklustre, it may be a sign that they need freshening up and recharging.

If you're using a crystal for protection, to support you through an illness or an emotionally heavy time, I'd suggest you cleanse it every day or at least once a week – you could use a crystal cluster, smudging or a crystal cleansing spray. Opaque crystals, like Malachite, which absorb more negative energy and pollution, need cleansing more often. Crystals that allow light to pass through them, like Clear Quartz or Herkimer Diamond, elevate energy into a higher frequency so they don't store as much negativity.

You could cleanse your crystals once a week, once a month or whenever the mood takes you. You could simply waft around some palo santo or spritz your crystal cleansing spray, or craft your own mass crystal cleansing ritual that's aligned with a specific moon phase, solstice or equinox.

Any time is a good time to show your crystals some TLC.

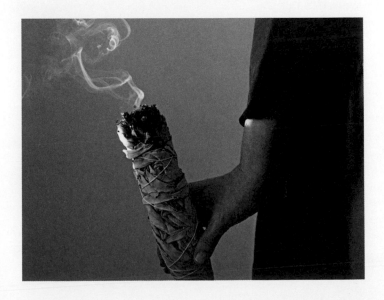

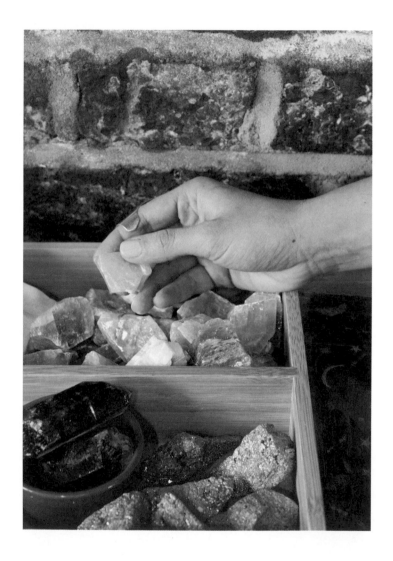

## CAN OTHER PEOPLE TOUCH MY CRYSTALS?

This is up to you. If you want to let someone hold your crystals, then go for it, and if you don't, you're more than entitled to decline. Some cultures would view crystals as sacred items and, if they're used for ceremonies and rituals, contact is reserved solely for the celebrant, which is totally cool. Some people worry that another person's 'negative' or 'bad' energy may rub off on a crystal and contaminate it: it's worth considering that other people's energy isn't necessarily good or bad, but some are just in need of an extra dose of compassion. Someone (like you) may be drawn to your crystal for a reason and may benefit from connecting with it. When we focus on the 'negative' aspects of another person (or situation) we may perpetuate that side of them; seeing them through the lens of kindness and compassion can create a radical shift in our relationship. Remember that crystals are highly intelligent so can recalibrate their energy accordingly, and you can always use the cleansing techniques described earlier in this chapter if you're concerned. If you aren't happy to share your crystals, you could either let the other person keep the crystal after they've held it (if appropriate), or if you don't want them to hold it, politely say, 'No.' If you're feeling generous, you could give them another crystal. It's important to feel into and do what's right for you.

'Remember that crystals are highly intelligent so can recalibrate their energy accordingly'

## HOW TO CHARGE YOUR CRYSTALS

**We all need a little boost sometimes! Think of how reinvigorated you feel after the sun has warmed your skin or when you're salty and fresh from swimming in the sea. Crystals *love* being energized by nature too.**

### Sunshine

Leave your crystal to soak up some sun rays for solar energy. Avoid leaving it in direct sunlight for too long: too much sunlight can fade the colour of some crystals and is also a potential fire risk with Quartz (in extreme cases it magnifies the sun's rays and starts a fire).

### Moonlight

Have you seen the 'I can't come out to tonight: I'm charging my crystals' meme that is usually shared on a full moon? I love knowing there's a time of the month when people are collectively showing their crystals some love, but it's good to know that you can charge your crystal under any phase of the moon. You can use each phase to support the intention for your crystal.

- New moon: new beginnings and ventures

- Waxing moon: inspiration, hope and optimism

- Full moon: abundance and celebration

- Waning moon: protection, detoxing and letting go of old relationships/habits/attachments

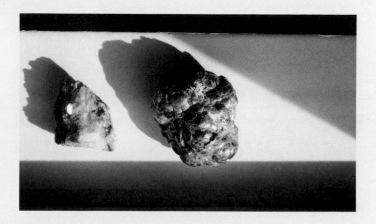

## Running water

Nothing beats coming home after a long slog and standing under the shower as it washes away the day. You step out feeling so fresh and clean. Running water can stimulate and elevate the energy of crystals too. If you wanted to multitask, you could take a few crystals into the shower with you or just leave them under running water – in the sink or in a stream (just be careful you don't lose your crystal). If you're leaving the crystal in the sink, put the plug in and allow the water to run until it covers the crystal, then leave the crystal to soak for an hour or overnight.

If you're near the beach, you could let gentle waves wash over your crystals to energize them. Again, hold them tightly so they aren't washed away.

Keep in mind that some crystals may be damaged when they come into contact with water, like Selenite, Pyrite, Lapis Lazuli, Haematite and Opal. If you happen to pass a river, or you're at the beach and you want to charge the crystal with some watery vibes, place them somewhere near to the water but dry.

## Earth

Allow your crystals to absorb Mother Earth's energies by placing them on the ground. You could try burying them but don't forget the treasure map to find them again.

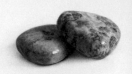

# 'I can't come out tonight...

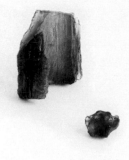

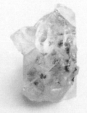

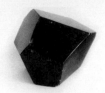
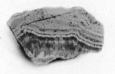
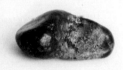

...I'm charging
my crystals'

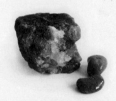
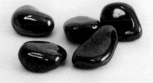

# HOW TO PROGRAMME YOUR CRYSTAL

After you've cleansed and charged your crystal, it's time to join forces with it. What do you want your crystal to help you with?

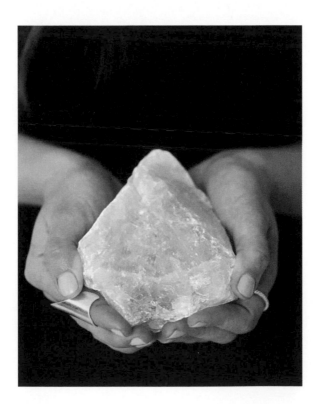

Is it to help you feel more confident/loved/energized/supported/to get over your ex/have a night of sweet dreams? Whatever the reason that this crystal has come into your life, it's great to communicate and share how you'd like to collaborate with it.

You may not feel called to programme the crystal with a specific intention and that's okay. It's important to trust that it's already perfectly aligned with you and will adapt to support your needs in each moment, sometimes regardless of your intention. If your crystal was given to you or found its way to you through synchronicity, you need not programme it because a higher intelligence may be at play.

When you're giving a crystal as a present, you can programme it on behalf of your friend. Think of why you chose it and how you'd like it to support that special someone.

## CRYSTAL PROGRAMMING

### Version 1

1.  Hold the crystal in both hands and imagine that you and the crystal are surrounded by pure white light.

2.  State your intention, either aloud or in your mind: 'I programme this crystal to support me in feeling more confident to set clear boundaries in my life/opening my heart to experiencing love/trusting my intuition/accepting myself/believing that I deserve all kinds of abundance [insert whatever you'd like to experience or feel more of] for the highest good of all. Thank you.'

### Version 2

1.  Hold the crystal in both hands and imagine that you and the crystal are surrounded by pure white light.

2.  Imagine your intention as a gold seed in your heart and visualize it growing until it becomes a flower (this can be any flower). As the flower becomes more vivid in your imagination, visualize a golden cord reaching from your heart through your arms and into the crystal in your hands. The gold cord is the connection between your intention and your crystal.

3.  State your intention, either aloud or in your mind: 'I programme this crystal to support me in feeling more confident to set clear boundaries in my life/opening my heart to experiencing love/trusting my intuition/accepting myself/believing that I deserve all kinds of abundance [insert whatever you'd like to experience or feel more of] for the highest good of all. Thank you.'

If you're looking for programming inspiration, try using this chart. Take a few moments to relax and close your eyes. Before you open them, ask: 'What would you like to have/experience/receive/feel?'

**When you open your eyes what word do you see first?**

| N | O | U | R | I | S | H | U | R | H | E | A | L | T | H |
|---|---|---|---|---|---|---|---|---|---|---|---|---|---|---|
| T | S | U | R | R | E | N | D | E | R | P | E | F | P | T |
| I | P | A | I | S | E | L | F | L | O | V | E | R | R | U |
| N | P | A | S | S | I | O | N | A | M | I | N | I | O | I |
| T | D | R | E | A | M | S | F | X | A | S | E | E | T | N |
| U | S | C | O | U | R | A | G | E | N | I | W | N | E | S |
| I | C | T | S | H | A | R | E | O | C | O | B | D | C | P |
| T | A | B | U | N | D | A | N | C | E | N | E | S | T | I |
| I | L | A | P | R | E | C | E | I | V | E | G | P | R | R |
| O | M | R | P | U | S | A | M | B | I | T | I | O | N | E |
| N | B | L | O | S | S | O | M | U | C | R | N | W | H | L |
| C | E | S | R | T | M | O | N | E | Y | U | N | E | O | E |
| G | R | A | T | I | T | U | D | E | H | S | I | R | M | A |
| A | D | V | E | N | T | U | R | E | R | T | N | A | E | S |
| S | C | R | E | A | T | E | M | F | O | R | G | I | V | E |

Once you've found your word/s, allow yourself some time to reflect on what it means to you. I'd suggest spending some time writing down any thoughts, ideas or feelings that arise from this task so that you can devise a programming statement that feels good for you.

## THE BONUS STEP

The next step, which a lot of people don't mention about crystals, is that *you* need to collaborate and play your part in this cosmic deal. You can place your crystals in all of the 'right' places but if you aren't taking action to support what you're asking for, you may be disappointed and another crystal will end up in a dusty trinket bowl, a.k.a. the crystal graveyard, because apparently it didn't do its job properly. You can't bypass the fact that it's ultimately your responsibility to bring this magic to life, not the crystal's.

Once you choose to work with a crystal, it's likely that situations will arise to serve as doorways for you to learn about yourself through its lens. This may seem like a challenge or a perfectly timed synchronicity. Both are affirmations that you're on the right track. Hello, transformation incoming!

Say yes to opportunities. Give yourself time and space to unravel limiting self-beliefs and make peace with your insecurities. Advocate for yourself, and give yourself permission to enforce boundaries around your time and energy. Most importantly, invest in yourself and believe that you deserve all kinds of wonderful. Crystals will help you to confront anything that's waiting to be healed.

# 'The secret to change is to focus all of your energy not on fighting the old but building the new'

### FROM *THE WAY OF THE PEACEFUL WARRIOR*, DAN MILLMAN

Take some time to consider why you chose the crystal and what resonates with you about its personality. How can you collaborate with the crystal and its wisdom to transform your situation and expand your life?

There's a reason why crystals find their way to us. They facilitate a healing process, but ultimately the life changes come from you. If you want changes in your life, you need to take action and become the master of your destiny.

# CONNECTING WITH YOUR CRYSTALS

**Every crystal has its own personality and can bring out something different in all of us. For example: we all have our own sense of humour and find different things engaging. I think Russell Brand is hilarious and fascinating but you may disagree.**

Someone may say that a crystal means something specific but that doesn't have to apply to you. In the workshops that I lead, twenty people may meditate with Amethyst and each person may gain a different impression of its personality. Every crystal has a distinguishing quality but a whole spectrum of feelings and experiences may be connected to it.

It's up to you to get to know your crystal and find out what it means to *you*.

**You can do this through meditation:**

- Sit in a quiet place where you won't be disturbed.

- Take a few deep breaths to centre your energy and bring your consciousness fully into the present moment.

- As you hold your crystal in your hand, with your eyes closed, visualize the crystal's energy travelling into your hands, through your arms, into your body and up into your head.

- Feel the crystal activating your third eye – the space between your eyebrows, in the middle of your forehead.

- As your crystal activates your third eye, feel yourself connected to the crystal.

- Feel yourself absorbing its healing energy.

- When you feel ready you can ask the crystal some questions.

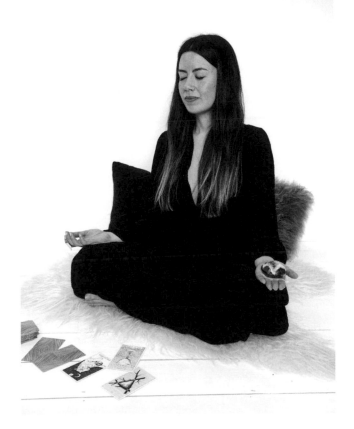

You could ask it what its name is and what healing energy it wants to share with you. You can ask it how you can best harness its powers and where it would like to be kept. How should it be used?

Take some time to get familiar with your crystal, just as you would when you make a new friend. Don't try to force answers from it. Initially you may get a word, a colour, a symbol or a feeling from it. Trust that it is sharing with you exactly what you need to know at this time. Getting to know your crystal better will come with practice but it's much more fun doing it this way than looking it up in this book or on the internet!

# CHAKRAS

**You may have heard chakras mentioned in a yoga or meditation class or by one of your 'witchy' or 'hippie' friends. We all have them. Chakras sprang from ancient eastern philosophies and healing practices, but the concept is used by many modern healers and teaching systems because of their relevance to our sense of well-being and health. The word 'chakra' is Sanskrit (an ancient eastern language) and means 'wheel' or 'disc'.**

There are seven fundamental chakras that act as invisible centres to support our life force: the root/base chakra, sacral chakra, solar plexus chakra, heart chakra, throat chakra, third eye/brow chakra and crown chakra. They're aligned vertically, beginning in the pelvic area and stacking up along the spine to the top of your head. Each chakra is represented by a colour and is associated with specific functions and empowerments.

The chakras are the unseen equivalent of the endocrine system and are often associated with each other. The endocrine system is a team of glands that work together, with a little help from your hormones. Your endocrine system is vital to regulating everything that you need to function: hormones, metabolism, growth and development, fertility, sleep, mood and so much more. If anything is out of sync, it's likely to affect your physical health and energy levels. When it comes to your energetic body, the aura and chakras are in charge of managing your vibes and keeping them flowing. Your aura is the electromagnetic field that emanates from the physical body and your chakras regulate how you move through life on an energetic level.

Our lives are in constant flux between balance and imbalance, reflected by the chakras. Although each chakra has its own function, they interact simultaneously, responding to and processing your thoughts, emotions and experiences. Understanding your chakras and how they work can help you identify any imbalances in your life: a useful tool for self-awareness and personal development.

For some people, the tight knot they feel in their stomach every Monday morning, which makes them so anxious that they swap breakfast for a double-shot coffee, is 'normal' or part of who they are. It may also be a mechanism that helps them survive their environment, which isn't always conducive to their overall health and happiness. That used to be me: I had symptoms of a solar plexus and root chakra imbalance. Just because you don't always notice an obvious reaction to stress or trauma doesn't mean you haven't been affected by it. On an energetic level there will always be some kind of impact – big or small, conscious or unconscious. Luckily, the state of your chakras will reveal what's going on behind the scenes.

Chakras are often diagnosed as 'blocked', which means that unprocessed feelings and experiences are obstructing their natural flow, like a slow puncture in a tyre: it keeps deflating no matter how many times you pump it up. A blocked chakra can manifest as anxiety, depression, low self-esteem, self-sabotage, physical illness or a story that keeps repeating in your life: you miss opportunities because you don't speak up for yourself or you gravitate towards undesirable situations because you don't trust your intuition. This doesn't mean there's anything wrong with you: these are just life lessons waiting to be realized. Sluggish chakras simply need an extra dose of TLC and a greater awareness of attachments or thought processes that you're outgrowing.

If one chakra is blocked, the others may overcompensate and hijack the show. For example, a wide-open heart chakra could lead you to give too much in relationships, with disregard for your own needs and desires. An overactive base chakra may result in your becoming too focused on money and career to the detriment of your personal relationships. A busy throat chakra may make you extra communicative with the truth bombs, while you forget to listen to others.

When it comes to happy chakras, it's all about balance. Equal amounts of give and take, work and play, action and surrender. Chakra care means placing positive boundaries around your time and energy so that if you need space to work out how you're feeling, or what you want from life, you've got it. You'll know when your chakras are aligned because you'll be in total flow with whatever comes your way: you'll be more resilient to stress and challenges with the confidence to say yes to all the things that support and nourish you.

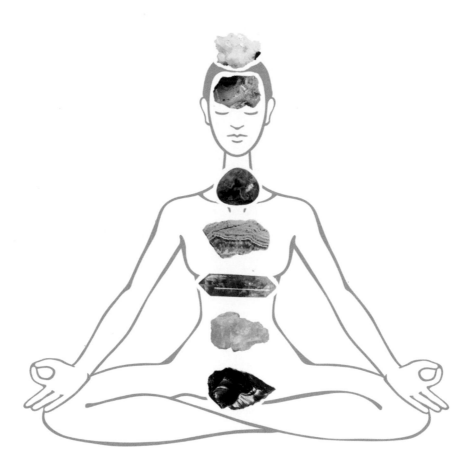

It's important to show all of your chakras love rather than favouring some over others – unless there's a chakra that's obviously in need of care and attention (this could be your root chakra if you're feeling run-down or anxious, the heart chakra if you're going through a break-up, the throat chakra if you've got laryngitis). Because the chakras correlate with the endocrine system you can remedy physical imbalances by working with crystals that are associated with a specific area. Like a machine, they are all equal components that work most efficiently when they're in synergy with each other.

Crystals are like superfoods for chakras, nourishing the energy as it flows through them. Crystals can support you to rewire your chakras and guide you towards feeling like the ultimate version of yourself. By using crystals to focus on specific chakras (or all of them) you can recharge, rebalance and awaken your innate superpowers.

## CRYSTALS FOR CHAKRAS

Choosing crystals based on their colour or chakra association will direct energy to this area of the body. I've included the traditional chakra associations for each crystal in my crystal guide (see pages 111–253) or you can use the diagram below as a quick guide. See it as a transport map: different colours represent the routes you can travel, and each line takes you to specific places. However, choose the crystals you're most drawn to, regardless of their traditional associations.

## HOW TO GET TO KNOW YOUR CHAKRAS BETTER

Choose seven crystals, one that represents each chakra, and for seven days meditate with each crystal in turn (Meditations, see page 64). I'd recommend beginning with the base chakra on the first day and working up to the crown chakra.

Use a pendulum (see page 81) regularly to check how your chakras are flowing. You could draw simple illustrations in a journal of the pendulum's movements; observe any patterns you notice using pens or pencils in the corresponding colours.

| | CHAKRA | COLOUR | FUNCTION | EMPOWERMENT |
|---|---|---|---|---|
| | CROWN | Violet | Spiritual connection, cosmic and divine consciousness, bliss | 'I understand' |
| | THIRD EYE | Indigo | Intuition, spiritual development, awareness | 'I see' |
| | THROAT | Blue | Communication, creative expression | 'I speak' |
| | HEART | Green/Pink | Love, trust, self-love, compassion, connection | 'I love' |
| | SOLAR PLEXUS | Yellow | Confidence, personal power, motivation | 'I do' |
| | SACRAL | Orange | Emotions, sexuality, creativity, family relationships | 'I feel' |
| | ROOT | Red | Grounding, stability, independence, career, health, security | 'I am' |

| ORGANS | GLANDS | CRYSTALS |
|---|---|---|
| Spinal cord, brainstem | Pineal – regulates biological cycles, including sleep | Clear Quartz, Apophyllite, Rainbow Moonstone, Opal |
| Eyes, brain, pituitary and pineal glands | Pituitary– produces hormones and governs the five lower glands. Also associated with pineal gland | Amethyst, Charoite, Lepidolite, Shattuckite |
| Respiratory system, mouth, bronchial tubes, vocal cords | Thyroid – regulates body temperature and metabolism | Lapis Lazuli, Blue Lace Agate, Chrysocolla |
| Heart, lungs | Thymus gland – regulates immune system | Rose Quartz, Kunzite, Rhodochrosite, Morganite |
| Intestines, liver, pancreas, upper spine, stomach, bladder | Pancreas –regulates metabolism | Citrine, Sunstone, Tiger's Eye, Pyrite |
| Ovaries, bladder, prostate, kidneys, gall bladder, bowel, spleen | Adrenal – regulates immune system and metabolism | Orange Calcite, Unakite, Aragonite, Carnelian |
| Testes, kidneys, spine | Reproductive – sexual development and secretes sex hormones | Smoky Quartz, Obsidian, Garnet, Haematite |

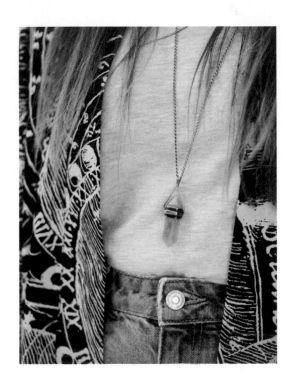

# NEVER FULLY DRESSED WITHOUT CRYSTALS

Not that we ever need an excuse to wear our crystals when they look so cool and are guaranteed to complete any #OOTD! If you want to upgrade from stashing your crystals in your bra or pockets, here are some ways that you can rock your crystals and wear them to supercharge your vibes.

## NECK

Make a statement and wear your treasures around your neck. What message do you want to send out to the universe? Actions speak louder with crystals. Wearing a crystal pendant can activate your chakras and protect your energy. A Rose Quartz pendant over your heart chakra may be a declaration of self-love or may proclaim that you're open only to the highest expressions of love: players aren't welcome. Wearing a piece of Citrine on a pendant long enough to float over your solar plexus chakra can help you stay plugged into your integrity and reinforce some much-needed boundaries.

## HANDS

According to palmistry we have the entire universe in our hands. The fingers and other areas of the hand are associated with different aspects of our personality, the five elements (air, water, fire, earth and ether/spirit) and the planets. Wearing your rings on specific fingers can activate an intention. Kundalini yogis are often seen wearing a ring on their Jupiter finger (or index finger). Jupiter is the planet associated with luck and expansion. Wearing a ring on this finger is said to enhance your sense of power and strengthen your leadership potential. The tradition of wearing a wedding ring on the fourth finger of the left hand dates from the Romans, who believed that the vein in it ran directly to the heart. It was known as the *vena amoris* – the vein of love. If you're choosing your engagement ring, or dropping subtle hints to your lover, perhaps you could choose a stone based on the energies that you'd like to flow into your relationship.

Yoga philosophies consider the left side of the body as feminine (intuitive, receiving, creative, flowing, nurturing) and the right as masculine (initiating, active, giving, assertive, constructive). We're all a unique blend of the two archetypal energies. With this in mind, you could wear your rings or bracelets based on the side of you you'd like to harness. While I've been writing this book, I've been wearing a Labradorite ring on the Saturn middle finger of my right hand: Saturn relates to discipline and the right hand (masculine) implies action; my intention is less procrastination, more manifestation.

When choosing which hand to wear your jewels on, you could think of the left as supporting what you'd like to invite into your life and receive, and the right as what you'd like to commit to or let go. Get curious with what magic you can activate by wearing your crystals on different fingers/hands to find out what works for you.

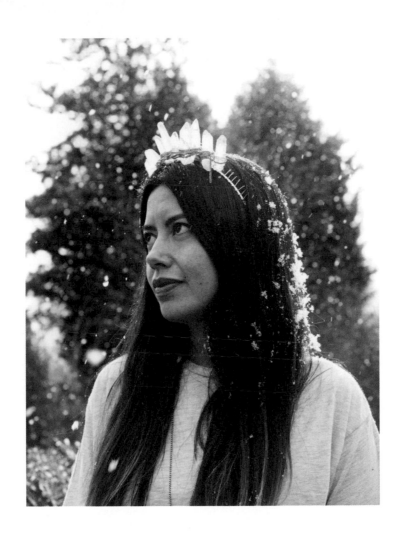

## WEAR THEM LIKE A QUEEN

Crystal headpieces don't have to be kept for special occasions. Activate your upper chakras, like the crown chakra and the third eye, by wearing a crystal crown, tiara or earrings. They can help you drop into a deeper meditation and channel spiritual energy.

# 'Activate your upper chakras, like the crown chakra and the third eye, by wearing a crystal crown'

In Vedic astrology gemstones are worn to enhance planetary influences. According to an ancient Hindu legend, they are associated with the demon king Bali, a devotee of the Lord Vishnu, who had blessed him with the gift of invincibility, which had enabled Bali to defeat all of the *devas* (gods) in battle. Although Bali was known as the king of demons, he was also renowned for his benevolence and generosity, which the gods knew to be his 'weak' spot. They knew they could use this to their advantage to reclaim power over Heaven. So, Indra, the god of Heaven, disguised himself as a priest and sought Bali to assist him in finding an animal for a sacrificial ceremony. Indra feigned desperation because he was running out of time: the ceremony couldn't be performed without the sacrifice. Bali, of course, wanted to help and transformed himself into a buffalo knowing that his body was invincible. As the gods gathered for the ceremony, Indra hurled his thunderbolt weapon (*vajra*) directly at Bali's head, knowing that it wasn't invincible, unlike his body. Bali had been tricked and because he'd offered himself out of pure altruism, his body parts shattered into precious gems. His bones became Diamonds, his teeth became Pearls, his blood became Rubies, his eyes became Blue Sapphires, his skin became Yellow and White Sapphires, his heart became Lapis Lazuli, his flesh became Coral, his bile became Emeralds, his fat became Quartz, and apparently the rest of his body became Agate. Each gemstone was claimed by a planet, which was why humans were guided to harness their powers to amplify the planets' resonance in their lives.

'According to palmistry we have the entire universe in our hands. The fingers and other areas of the hand are associated with different aspects of our personality, the five elements (air, water, fire, earth and ether/spirit) and the planets'

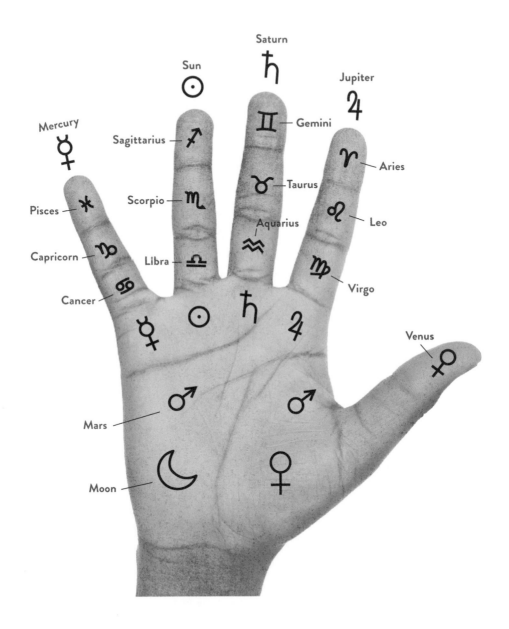

Mercury

Sun

Saturn

Jupiter

Sagittarius

Gemini

Aries

Pisces

Scorpio

Taurus

Leo

Capricorn

Aquarius

Libra

Cancer

Virgo

Venus

Mars

Moon

# CRYSTAL SHAPES

Every crystal's personality can be influenced by its shape, whether it's a natural formation or mechanically treated through shaping and polishing. Some people prefer crystals in their natural form, considering it the organic and most potent version. Others believe that 'enhancing' crystals diminishes their powers. Treating crystals may offer additional benefits, such as revealing otherwise-hidden beauty and patterns, and focusing the direction of energy. Raw versus polished: which do you prefer?

## GEODE

From the outside geodes appear to be ordinary rocks until they're cracked open to reveal a surprise cave of glistening crystals. They're the Kinder Eggs of the crystal realm! Geodes are available to purchase as sets that include a geode rock and a small hammer for you to discover what's hidden inside.

## PYRAMID

Pyramids are stones that have been shaped to have four equal triangular sides with a square base. They can be used to amplify energy and intentions, which is great for crystal grids, healing work and manifesting spells.

## CLUSTERS

Crystal clusters, like Clear Quartz, Amethyst and Apophyllite, bring harmony to the home and workplace: they represent collaboration and teamwork.

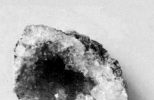

Geode

Pyramid

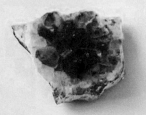

Clusters

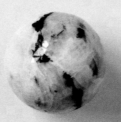

Sphere

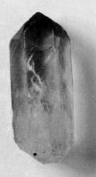

Double
Terminated

Natural
Point

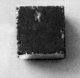

Square

Tumbled

## SPHERE

Most of us are familiar with the archetypal image of a fortune teller and their crystal ball. When a crystal is shaped into a sphere, it can be used for scrying – taking a peek into the past or future. Crystal spheres will emit energy equally in all directions, which is why they're perfect for scrying: they enable you to see a situation from all angles.

## NATURAL POINT

In this form the crystal is faceted at one point and can be used to focus energy. If you direct the point towards you it will draw energy to you, and if you direct it away it will draw energy away from you. Large natural crystal points, like those in Clear Quartz, can be used as wands to activate other crystals and healing grids.

## DOUBLE TERMINATED

When a crystal has a point at each end it is known as double terminated. Crystals can be cut and polished into this shape or they form naturally, as with Herkimer Diamonds. These crystals simultaneously attract and emit energy, which is ideal for balancing polarities. If you're the kind of person who's always give-give-giving and not so comfortable with asking for help, or if you find it hard to feel present in the here and now, this shape's for you. They can be used for healing grids and meditation.

## SQUARE

Square crystal can be shaped or forms naturally, as in Pyrite. This formation is good for grounding and bringing stability to a situation.

## TUMBLED

Tumbled crystals have been smoothed and polished, transformed from their raw formation. They're often placed inside a 'rock tumbler' so that any rough edges can be smoothed away. Tumbled stones are thought of as the most understated of crystal formations because they're affordable and easily attainable. They're the perfect travel companions, fit discreetly into your pockets and can be used for grids and meditations.

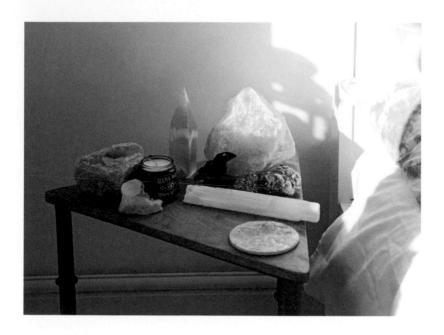

# WHERE TO KEEP
# YOUR CRYSTALS

**While crystals will undoubtedly add extra sparkle to a room, placing them in specific areas of your home and workspace will encourage the good vibes to keep flowing.**

### BEDROOM

Turn your bedroom into a sanctuary with crystals. A few, mindfully placed, can infuse it with calming energies that will help to fade the stresses of your day and press pause on everything that can wait until tomorrow. Selenite is an ideal crystal to have in your bedroom because it gently harmonizes the energy of the space and creates a relaxing atmosphere. If you're struggling to sleep at night, and counting sheep doesn't work for you, keep a piece of Lepidolite under your pillow or beside your bed. Its soothing energy will help you to feel grounded and slow down your overactive mind so that you can drift into a night of sweet dreams. Other crystals that support a good night's sleep are Moonstone, Amethyst, Black Tourmaline and Celestite.

Looking for a love spell? According to *feng shui* practices, if you keep two pieces of Rose Quartz together by the bed, you'll attract harmonious and loving relationships – you could also try this with Cobalto Calcite or Kunzite. Want more passion? Place a piece of Garnet, Orange Calcite or Ruby at each corner of the bed to create a mini grid (see page 77): these fiery crystals may ignite the spark you've been missing.

## KITCHEN

The kitchen may seem like an unusual place to keep your crystals, and while they obviously aren't edible and won't burn calories, they can have a positive influence on what we choose to consume. Amethyst and Tiger's Eye are a dynamic duo when it comes to cultivating new habits and overcoming temptation, especially when you're detoxing or slaying a sugar addiction.

## WORKPLACE

On days when life feels like one huge procrastination and you're surrounded by distractions, call on your crystals to get your eyes focused on the prize again. Crystals like Pyrite, Rutilated Quartz, Red Jasper, Labradorite and Carnelian offer us some much-needed grounding energy so that we can tune into what really needs to be done and increase productivity. If you're spending a lot of time on your phone, laptop or computer, or you work with electrical equipment, keep Galena, Black Tourmaline, Smoky Quartz and Malachite close by to absorb any electromagnetic pollution or radiation that the devices emit. Electrical equipment creates positive ions, which may cause you to feel overwhelmed, lethargic, anxious and stressed. Black Tourmaline is a hero when it comes to neutralizing ions and helping you find your way back to the flow lane.

Teamwork and cooperation can be the key to success when it comes to projects. A Clear Quartz cluster or Spirit Quartz will encourage a united force, and Septarian may boost your ability to collaborate successfully with others.

## BATHROOM

Transform your bathroom into an oasis for your ritual baths/showers (see page 104) by using crystals to enhance the ambience. One of my favourite crystals to keep in the bathroom is Rose Quartz: it's a reminder of the importance of self-care and self-love. It is famous for its nurturing personality and encourages us to be kind to ourselves and others. It guides us to be less critical of what we see in the mirror because beauty really does come in all shapes and sizes.

# CHAPTER TWO

# CRYSTAL RITUALS

# MEDITATING
# WITH CRYSTALS

Spirituality and meditation are the heartbeat of my self-care practice. Connecting with myself like this every day nurtures a deeper sense of self-awareness and supports me to feel more grounded. I make sure that I stop, drop and meditate, especially in times of stress or when I'm feeling overwhelmed. It never fails to make me feel that I'm flowing with the universe again.

Meditation is proven to reduce stress and anxiety, maximize good vibes, encourage positive habits, increase focus and motivation, improve sleep quality and boost confidence, to name but a few of the many benefits. It's never been easier to get into meditation because there's a plethora of ways in which you can tune in to tune out, from chanting mantras, listening to guided meditations, colouring mandalas to taking a mindful walk in nature. It can be as simple as downloading a meditation app, putting on your headphones and giving yourself ten minutes of calm while you're on the train to work – this is my favourite kind of multitasking. Every method of meditation leads to the same place: calling back the wandering thoughts that have complicated the simplest things so that you can learn how to flow with whatever life throws at you. As I took a break from writing this, I saw a (synchronistic) meme saying, 'Did you know that 10–20 minutes of meditation per day can significantly reduce your risk of giving a shit?' Amen to that.

Occasionally, when the subject of meditation comes up in conversation, I'm met with an array of reasons why someone can't meditate. It often goes something like this: 'I wish I could meditate *but* . . . I don't have enough time/I'm too busy/I can't sit still for that long/I can't switch my mind off/I've tried it once but I thought it was boring/it's too hard/don't you have to be a Buddhist to meditate?' My answer: 'Meditation is a *practice*.' If you choose to give meditation a chance and persist, you will find your own rhythm. There's no right (or wrong) way to do it. Meditation is an accumulation of moments in which you dedicate your focus to something that supports you – it's much easier when it feels alluring, rather than a chore or something else to tick off your never-ending to-do list.

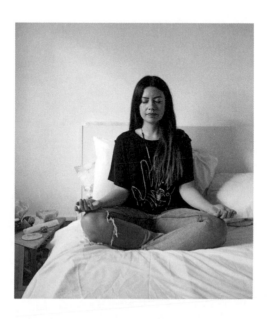

You've got to want to meditate. Try something that feels good and inspiring to you. It could be a guided meditation, chanting, mantras, vedic or transcendental meditation, yoga, painting, gardening, mandalas or walking a labyrinth. You can do it anywhere: in bed, on your yoga mat, in the bath, on the beach, in the garden, on the bus – anywhere you can create a nook and not be disturbed, anywhere that makes you feel comfortable to tune out from your usual distractions. If you're able to kill time scrolling, you aren't too busy to meditate. If you've got time to press snooze a few times on your morning alarm, you could swipe to listen to a meditation instead of pressing it again. If you can binge-watch the latest must-see series on TV, you can sit still for at least five minutes to meditate. And what better way to wrap up your day than with a dreamy meditation to decompress before you go to sleep? Then you can really start fresh tomorrow.

I used to be a self-confessed obsessive and over-thinker. If I can meditate, I honestly believe that anyone can.

Let me share a secret with you. When I first started learning how to meditate, I thought I was the worst 'meditator' *ever*. There I was in my bedroom, candles lit and incense burning, listening to a recording of a lady's soothing voice guiding me through a meditation. Instead of 'letting my thoughts drift away', all I could see was a wolf. It was quite frustrating and confusing. While I was supposed to be 'emptying' my thoughts, animals kept popping into my consciousness. It wasn't until later that I learnt they were spirit animals – in shamanism, spirit animals represent archetypal personalities that offer wisdom. That's how my alias became Wolf Sister. It was because I was relaxed that I was open to an alternative channel of awareness: meditation unlocked my intuition and allowed me to see these visions. Instead of being resistant to or angry about those thoughts, I was curious. When you tune out from external distractions, a gold mine of wisdom is waiting in your subconscious for you to explore. You'll find the answers that you're looking for when you stop and listen to yourself. Your practice doesn't have to be the same as mine or anybody else's. Taking time out (even if it's only a few minutes each day) to do something meditative is an opportunity to tune out of the hustle of everyday life so that you can connect with what you need. Slowing your thoughts enough to feel into the spaces between is where you'll find clarity. It's like pressing ctrl-alt-delete for the soul.

## WANT TO UPGRADE YOUR MEDITATION? ADD SOME CRYSTALS TO YOUR PRACTICE

Crystals can be used to amplify your meditation and self-care practice. During my crystal workshops, we often use crystals to meditate with, and people always say how much easier it is to relax into the practice and slow down their thoughts when they're using a crystal. Especially those who usually struggle to meditate. It's as if the crystals anchor you in the moment so that you can receive what you need. Choosing a specific crystal can support you in focusing on a theme or intention, and as you meditate with it, you'll start to align with its energy (see Entrainment, page 22).

The first time I meditated with a crystal, I was filled with an intoxicating sense of lucidity and inspiration. My mind was blown in all of the best ways. In my mid-twenties I went to see a colour therapist in an attempt to cure my anxiety. She had me gaze into a crystal ball on a light-box that projected a spectrum of colours. As I softened my focus to tune into the inclusions of the orb, everything slowed down and I felt a profound connection with the crystal. All of the things that had been spinning me out before that moment became irrelevant. Y'know that feeling when you're blissed out after a massage, in no hurry to go anywhere fast? That is what happens when you meditate with crystals.

Meditating with your crystals can support you in overcoming anxiety and addictions, help you to heal from traumas, enhance your psychic abilities, invoke inspiration and creativity, promote lucid dreaming and nurture a deeper sense of love, compassion and confidence. Meditating with crystals won't make your problems magically disappear but the crystals will guide you to see your situation with a fresh perspective. Then you can begin to untangle your thoughts and find a way to evolve beyond the cycle that you're in.

Crystals for meditation: Clear Quartz, Amethyst, Celestite, Apophyllite, Danburite, Selenite, Opal, Hypersthene, Angel Aura, Morganite.

# '. . . stop, drop and meditate'

# HOW TO MEDITATE WITH CRYSTALS

**Meditating with crystals need not be complicated. All you need is one crystal,\* or a few, and to be somewhere comfortable that you won't be disturbed. If you like, light some incense or use some of your favourite essential oils, put on some chill-out music, set a timer for how long you'd like to be in the crystal vortex, and get ready to relax.**

## SITTING UP

- Sit upright with your back straight and supported.

- Hold the crystal in your left hand.

- Close your eyes and simply focus on the natural movement of your breathing. Tune into your body and how it moves as you breathe in and out for a few moments, drifting with each breath.

- Connect with the crystal in your left hand and imagine its energy begin to flow into your hand, moving up through your arm and into your body.

- Visualize the crystal's energy flowing through your body, sensing the colour(s) spreading down to your feet, gradually moving across your shoulders all the way to your right hand and reaching up to the top of your head. Visualize your entire body radiating with this crystallized colour.

- Imagine your body absorbing the colour and the crystal's energy.

- Spend as long as you need in this meditation. You could continue to imagine the colours, focus on your breathing or simply allow yourself to be fully present in the moment without having to rush anywhere.

- When you're ready, start to tune into the sensations of your body, wriggle your fingers and toes, move your head from side to side, take a stretch and physically feel the crystal in your hand.

- Slowly become aware of your surroundings and open your eyes.

- Be gentle with yourself as you carry on with your day.

## LYING DOWN

- Make yourself comfortable. Lie flat on your back, either on your bed or a yoga mat.

- Place the crystal on your forehead (third eye chakra).

- Close your eyes and simply focus on the natural movement of your breathing. Tune into your body and how it moves as you breathe in and out for a few moments, drifting with each breath.

- Imagine the energy of your crystal begin to flow into your forehead, moving through your head and into your body.

- Visualize the crystal's energy drifting through your body, imagining the colour(s) spreading down to your feet, gradually moving across your shoulders, all the way to your hands and reaching back up to the top of your head. Visualize your entire body radiating with this crystallized colour.

- Imagine your body absorbing the colour and the crystal's energy.

- Spend as long as you need in this meditation. You could continue to imagine the colours, focus on your breathing or simply allow yourself to be fully present in the moment without having to rush anywhere.

- When you're ready, start to tune into the sensations of your body, wriggle your fingers and toes, remove the crystal from your forehead, move your head from side to side and take a stretch.

- Slowly become aware of your surroundings and open your eyes.

- Be gentle with yourself as you carry on with your day.

* Cleanse and programme your crystals before beginning this meditation (see pages 27 and 38)

# CHAKRA HEALING MEDITATION

**Choose seven crystals to represent each chakra. (See the chart on page 48 for suggestions or be guided by your intuition.)**

- Cleanse, charge and programme the crystals (as a group or individually).

- Create a Zen den where you can lie down comfortably without being disturbed – make sure you've got some cosy layers in case you get cold. Put your phone on silent so that you aren't interrupted. Choose some relaxing music to play in the background and set a timer for how long you'd like to chill with your crystals. I'd recommend twenty to sixty minutes.

- Before you place each crystal on the chakra position, rub it between your hands to activate it.

- Lie down and place your crystals. I'd recommend beginning at the root chakra, then your sacral, solar plexus, heart, throat, third eye and the crown – they're less likely to roll off your body if you place them in this order!

- Close your eyes and begin to relax.

- Take three slow, deep breaths.

- Begin to visualize each chakra activating. Imagine the crystal's colour seeping into the chakra it's connected to. As the crystal joins forces with the chakra, visualize the chakra's colour becoming brighter and more vivid.

- Connect with each crystal and chakra in the same way. This could be in sequence from crown to root chakra, vice versa, or in a random order.

- Once all of the chakras are activated, imagine a rainbow radiating throughout your body and invite the colours to flow wherever they want to go.

- Spend as long as you like absorbing these colours and relaxing in this space.

- When you're ready to finish, gradually become aware of your surroundings. Then take three slow breaths, stretch, and tune into the sensations of your body; wriggle your fingers and toes.

- Remove the crystals, beginning at the top of your head. Gather the crystals in the opposite direction in which you placed them. Disconnect from the energy of each crystal and express gratitude to it as you remove it from your body.

- Ground yourself: you can do this by stretching, rubbing your hands together, massaging your feet, walking barefoot on grass and/or eating some root vegetables.

- Before you carry on with your day, take some time to record your experience.

- Cleanse the crystals after the meditation and keep them close to you for the next twenty-four hours.

- Feel free to note down any insights that may have come to you during the meditation.

Drink plenty of water and be gentle with yourself for the next few hours as you integrate the energy you've channelled.

# CREATE YOUR CRYSTAL ALTAR

**They say that rolling stones gather no moss. Well, I've had my fair share of places to call home over the years, and I've created an altar in each. Altars are also one of my ritual elements in setting up for the ceremonies and workshops I lead. Wherever I've been, or whatever my situation, mindfully curating my latest go-to crystals, with other natural elements and inspirational objects, to make an altar acts as a path to anchoring my intentions and makes me feel more centred.**

An altar is an intentional space that pays homage to aspirations, memories and purpose. It can be somewhere that you celebrate your achievements and whatever you're grateful for. It can also be an expression of your creativity, hopes, dreams and passions. Although lots of cultures use altars, in temples, churches or shrines, to worship deities and honour religious or spiritual practices, anyone can have one. An altar becomes a focal point in your home (or wherever you choose to set yours up), which can enhance your connection with crystals and represent experiences you're inviting into your life. Treat it like a 3D vision board that evolves over time. A vision board is usually a collage of pictures, photos and inspiring quotes that depict your aspirations. You can use your altar in the same way. It can be elaborate or minimalist. It can be aligned with the seasons, solstices, equinoxes or moon phases. Your altar is a reflection of you and can take whatever form feels appropriate to you.

Before you gather the items for your crystal altar, consider: What crystals do you feel most drawn to use? What is your focus or intention? What do you want to manifest/experience/celebrate/honour? How do you want to feel when you're at your altar?

## LOCATION

Your altar can be somewhere in your home – bedroom, bathroom, living room, garden, workspace – or a place in nature (use organic items that leave no trace if you choose to go outdoors). It can be as big or small as you like. Ideally, your altar will be in a place where it won't be disturbed and you can sit there comfortably without distractions.

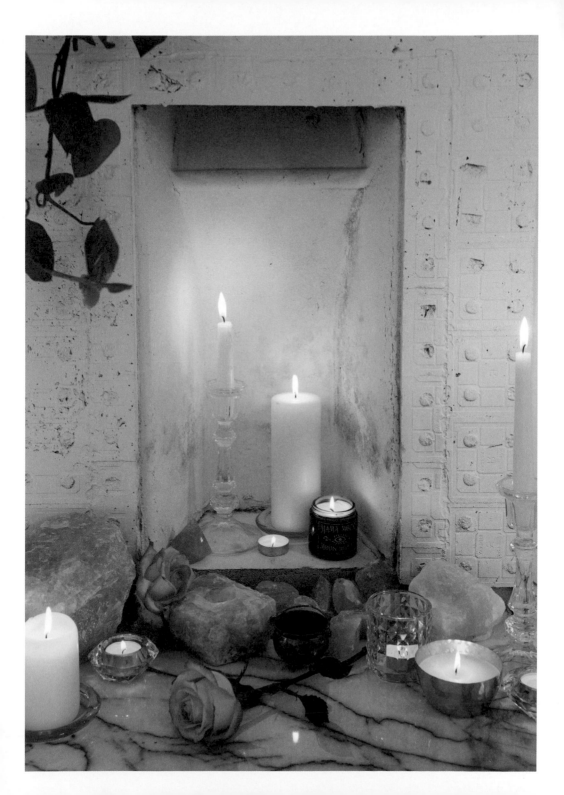

## CLEANSE

Make sure that the area is clutter-free and clean. Prepare the altar space by energetically purifying the area; you can do this with sage, palo santo or use the crystal cleansing spray (see page 108) in the same way that you would cleanse a crystal (page 27). Open a window and use a flame to light your sage or palo santo, let it burn a little, then allow the smoke to wash over your altar space. Having the window open allows the smoke to be ventilated and any unwanted energy can be released through the window.

## GATHER

Choose one or a few crystals* to activate your altar. You could also include totems, figurines, trinkets, souvenirs from your adventures or favourite holidays, flowers, plants, seashells, feathers, candles, incense, photographs, printed affirmations or quotes, postcards, artwork by your favourite creatives, poems, magazine cut-outs or oracle cards. Choose things you love that inspire you. You don't need to go on a huge spending spree to adorn your altar: you can use items that you already have at home or forage in nature for seasonal offerings.

## CREATE

Mindfully place each item on your altar; take your time to arrange things until they feel as if they're where they need to be. It can be simple, symmetrical, flamboyant, understated, overstated, colourful or monochrome. Express yourself and your intentions through your altar.

## CONNECT

Once you've finished setting up your altar, take some time to sit in front of it and connect with what you've created. You could meditate with the crystals from your altar and check in with how this space makes you feel. Record any insights, thoughts or feelings that came to you while performing this ritual. Your altar is a space where you can come to meditate, gather your thoughts and find inspiration.

All of these suggestions are adaptable and you're encouraged to create your altar in a way that you feel intuitively guided to.

---

\* Cleanse and programme your crystals before you place them on the altar (see pages 27 and 38). You can also do this with the other items for your altar, if you feel guided to.

## PORTABLE ALTAR

If you're staying away from home or travelling, I'd recommend taking a small selection of crystals and totems with you so that you feel relaxed and protected in unfamiliar surroundings. Choosing crystals to take away with me is the hardest part of my packing: I always take a small selection of tumbled stones, some palo santo, matches and a tea-light candle. When I've arrived at my destination, I'll set up my mini altar by the bed I'm going to be sleeping in. I'll add flowers or shells that I find while I'm out exploring during my stay.

Some people find it unsettling to sleep somewhere other than their own bed. If this applies to you, choose Selenite, Lepidolite and/or Amethyst. Turquoise and Aquamarine help to ensure safe travel, while Smoky Quartz and Black Tourmaline will help you feel grounded and protect your energy while you're in transit. If you're someone who finds travelling overwhelming, Moonstone will support you in going with the flow and feeling less stressed. If you're travelling long-haul, Haematite is the one for jet lag. And for those with a fear of flying, choose Tiger's Eye or Sardonyx.

# 'An altar acts as a path to anchoring my intentions and makes me feel more centred'

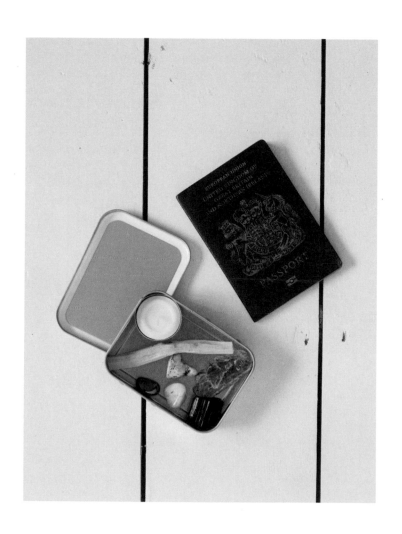

# CRYSTAL GRIDS

**Creating a crystal grid is a mindful ritual that will focus your attention and serves as a powerful way to unite crystals for a specific purpose. Crystal gridding can be used to activate all kinds of intentions, whether for self-love, to get over an ex, to overcome a social-media addiction or as a prayer for world peace.**

Use your crystal grid to envisage whatever inspires you. Grids usually have a basic symmetry, and some patterns incorporate sacred geometry. You can create your own patterns and experiment with layouts. There are no rules, no right or wrong way to set up your grid, so allow your intuition to be your guide.

## Crystals* needed

Crystal wand, large Quartz point or Selenite wand (to activate grid)

Crystal points or Selenite lasers

Tumbled stones or crystals

## Here are some ideas to create your own crystal grid

It can be as big or small as you like and the creative possibilities are endless. Arrange your grid on your altar (see page 72), or under your bed to improve your sleep. Place crystals in the corners of your room or throughout your home to bring good vibes to it and protect it from unwanted energies. Put them around the edges of your shower base, in your garden or on top of your vision board. I often place crystals around my yoga mat and lie within the boundaries of the crystal grid to receive its healing frequencies.

Start by either writing your intention or goal on a piece of paper, or choosing an oracle card or a picture of something that represents the purpose of your grid. Place it in the centre.

* As always, cleanse and programme your crystals before you use them (see pages 27 and 38).

I like to have a central crystal that signifies the main intention; the crystals placed around it act as the supporting energies that I'd like to help me. You could think of it like this: the main crystal is the lead singer of the band and the surrounding crystals are the backing singers, musicians and dancers.

Small crystal points can be used to direct energy in, out or around the grid, depending on how you place them. You could work with Clear Quartz for clarity, focus and to boost the other crystals; Amethyst for calming energy and to support spiritual intentions; Citrine to inspire action and confidence. Directing the crystal points inwards represents inner strength, supports and invites new opportunities to come to you; directing the crystal points outwards represents releasing attachments, habits and outdated beliefs, and may also signify generosity and sending out energy to others. Double terminated crystals (see page 59), like Herkimer Diamonds, will simultaneously direct energy in and out, representing balance and equality. Remember: you can attribute whatever significance to the positions feels good for you. These are just suggestions.

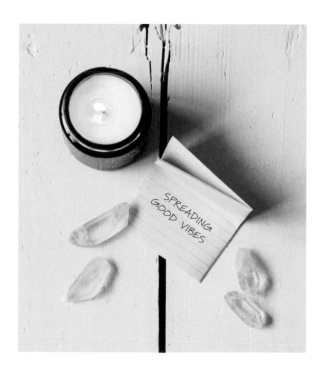

If you have just a few crystals, you could use three tumbled stones or crystal points to create a triangle layout. Direct the point towards you to invoke energy or point away from you to release energy.

You can use a larger Quartz point or crystal wand to activate the crystals. Touch each crystal with the crystal wand and imagine you're drawing lines of energy or weaving a golden thread that connects all of the crystals on the grid. Think: you're connecting the dots.

To give your crystal grid extra power, do this ritual on a new moon and keep it set up until the next full moon (or longer).

## SIMPLE CRYSTAL GRID

- Write your intention or an affirmation on a piece of paper. You could also use a tarot card that you'd like to work with or choose a picture that represents your vision.

- Place a crystal pyramid (see page 56) or a large crystal on the paper; this will be the centre point of your grid.

- Lay four Clear Quartz points or Selenite lasers around the crystal pyramid. Place them in the directions of north, east, south and west, with the points facing outwards.

- Place four crystals or tumbled stones between each of the Clear Quartz points.

- Using a crystal wand, touch the crystal pyramid, then touch the Clear Quartz point facing north. Imagine that you're joining their energy together. Repeat this step with each crystal that surrounds the crystal pyramid. Then touch the Clear Quartz point facing north and connect the other points and tumbled stones (work clockwise) as if you were connecting the dots to draw a circle around the crystal pyramid, finishing back at the Clear Quartz point facing north to complete the circle.

- Either spend some time meditating on your intention and visualize it coming to fruition or say your affirmation (aloud) three times.

- Express gratitude to the crystals for their support and blessings.

Crystals can work in mysterious ways and just because life shifts in a direction you didn't expect, it doesn't necessarily mean that the crystal/grid/intention/ritual hasn't worked. Sometimes letting go of old attachments happens quicker than you expected, but if it's happening, it means that you're ready. Sometimes the effects are so subtle, it's as if they take place right under your nose but it's not until later that you have the epiphany. Surrender. Trust the process. Expect something wonderful, with possible detours that will lead you to something even better than you could imagine.

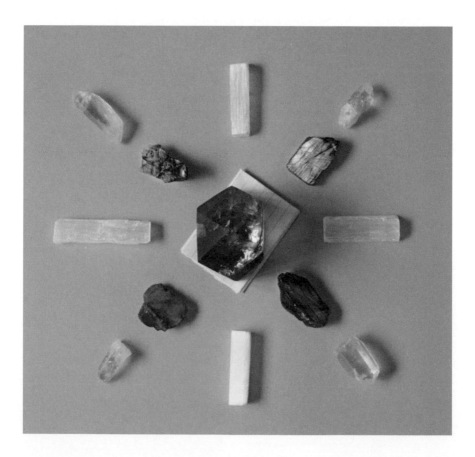

# DOWSING WITH A CRYSTAL PENDULUM

## WHAT IS A PENDULUM?

Pendulums are well-known tools for divination and dowsing. They're simple devices: a small weighted, symmetrical object that's suspended from a chain, cord or thread. In this book we'll be talking about crystal pendulums but you can also craft a pendulum with a ring, bead, trinket, key or even a paperclip, attached to some silk thread.

## WHAT ARE PENDULUMS USED FOR?

Pendulums love to answer questions – like Siri of the Now Age – and to support you in making decisions. Perhaps the best-known way to use the power of the pendulum is in predicting the gender of an unborn baby, traditionally done with a gold ring and thread. These days a lot of people seem to find out at their ultrasound scan whether they're having a boy or girl, but for some, who've decided to wait until she or he arrives, using the pendulum is a fun way to see if it can get it right.

I mostly use my pendulum in healing rituals to assess and balance my client's energy system. It will show me how the chakras are functioning and help to bring them into alignment. I also use the pendulum when doing tarot readings to clarify some of the messages. The pendulum is such a diverse tool and can even give your memory a little nudge when you need it: I can never remember what time I was born, which is actually really useful to know when you're doing your birth chart in astrology. So, I use my pendulum to find out. I start by asking, 'Was I born at one a.m.?', 'Was I born at two a.m.?', 'Was I born at three a.m.?' and so forth, noting the responses as I go along until I finally ask, 'Was I born at midnight?' Out of all the times, my pendulum only ever circles (yes) once, to remind me that I was born at ten p.m. It remains static for the twenty-three other times.

There are so many possibilities when it comes to pendulum dowsing. Here are a few more suggestions.

- To choose crystals

- To help you find lost items, pets or people

- To find water and ley lines

- To communicate with spirit energy, spirit guides and angels

## HOW DO PENDULUMS WORK?

The pendulum will translate the wisdom of your subconscious mind through motion; as it responds to your question the answer is represented by movement. Consider the mind–spirit connection: the aura and physical body are constantly processing energy and information, whether from your thoughts, feelings, experiences or other influences. In the same way that you might blush when you receive a compliment, laugh when you hear something funny or cry when you're upset, the body's reflexes respond to what's going on around you. Sometimes these responses are internalized and the impact of a situation isn't always immediately obvious. Even if you haven't noticed a physical reaction to what's happening around you, your aura and body will be processing the information.

The body is so wise and can reveal so much when you take the time to listen to it. When you attune to the pendulum it will amplify responses within the body that would usually be too subtle to see – in a similar way to using a speaker to listen to your music for higher quality and volume.

Ultimately, the answers are channelled from your highest self into a physical expression via the pendulum.

# 'The body is so wise and can reveal so much when you take the time to listen to it'

## HOW TO CHOOSE YOUR PENDULUM

Crystal pendulums are available from mystical shops and via the internet. Some people prefer Clear Quartz or Apophyllite pendulums because of their association with clarity and connecting with higher consciousness. My pendulum is made of Amethyst and I've had it for more than ten years. Unfortunately I dropped it a while ago and the tip broke off. I've tried to replace it with other pendulums, because of its apparent flaw, but the Amethyst is still my most trusted pendulum, the one I use time and time again. The same principles apply as they do for choosing a crystal (see page 23): be guided by the pendulum you feel most drawn to. It could be for its aesthetics, because it's your favourite crystal or just because it felt like *the one* and you didn't want to put it down.

## GETTING TO KNOW YOUR PENDULUM

As with any crystal, it's important to cleanse, charge and programme your pendulum with an intention before you use it. The intention could be something like 'I'm open to knowing the truth for the highest good of all' or 'May this pendulum reveal what I need to know for healing and inspiration.'

When you first start practising with your pendulum, I'd recommend sitting on a chair at a table. Sit upright with your back supported, shoulders relaxed and both feet firmly planted on the floor. Make sure that your hands and legs aren't crossed so that your energy can flow freely.

Hold the pendulum in your left or right hand – experiment with what feels most comfortable. Have the chain or thread of your pendulum between your thumb and index (first) finger – some pendulums have a small ring or hoop at the top of the chain to place your finger through to make it easier to hold the pendulum without using too much pressure. Support your arm by resting your elbow on the table as you hold the pendulum in front of you.

Suspend the pendulum high enough that it does not touch the table and has enough space to move freely. The opposite hand should be placed palm down on the table.

If you'd prefer to stand while working with your pendulum, make sure that you're standing straight with your elbow at a ninety-degree angle, your forearm parallel to the floor or ground.

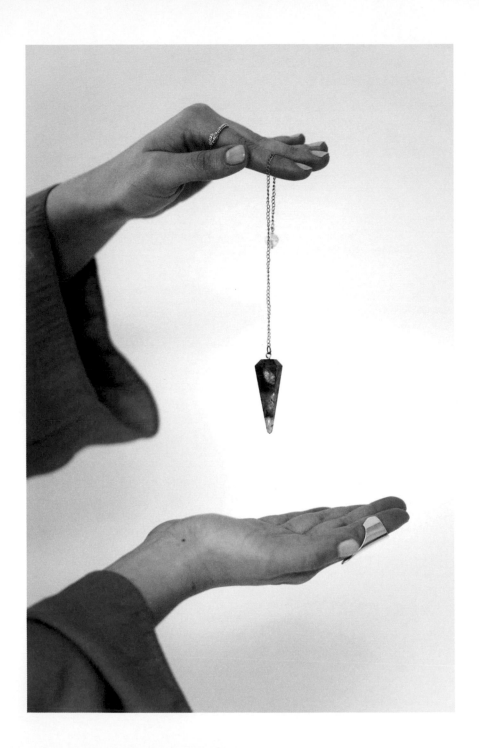

'Pendulums love to
answer questions – like Siri
of the Now Age – and to
support you in making
decisions'

Take a few moments to centre yourself and focus your attention on the pendulum. A simple way to do this would be to take three slow breaths: inhale deeply and extend the exhale to relax your body and calm your mind.

When working with the pendulum, specific yes or no questions are best. Due to its limited vocabulary (movements), the pendulum isn't adept at going into details such as how, why, what or when. There are usually four answers: yes, no, maybe, or I don't want to answer. The pendulum will respond by moving in different directions.

Start getting to know your pendulum by finding out what its movements represent for you – this varies between pendulums and people. Allow the pendulum to become still before you start asking questions and before each new question. Ask (in your mind or out loud) questions to which you know the answers so that you can decipher the responses: Am I female? Am I male? Is my name . . .? Am I . . . years old? Have fun with the questions. Alternatively you could ask it to show you its directions for 'yes', 'no', 'maybe' and 'I don't know'. Make a note of what the movements represent. Take your time to get used to how your pendulum moves and be patient: sometimes it can take a little while for your pendulum to warm up. Anyone can use a pendulum, but you have to be open and relaxed.

Once you're familiar with the movements for the four answers, you can ask questions to which you *really* want to know the answers.

It's important to use the pendulum when you're relaxed and have a meditative mindset to allow the most accurate answers to be channelled. Your desire for a specific outcome can override the natural movement of the pendulum so it's important to detach yourself from what you *want* to see. Consciously set the intention to step aside from your ego so that the pendulum will show you the truth. Keep this in mind if you have a strong emotional attachment to a question – I'd suggest waiting until you feel more detached from it, or ask someone impartial to hold the pendulum for you.

'Make a note of what the movements represent. Take your time to get used to how your pendulum moves and be patient: sometimes it can take a little while for your pendulum to warm up. Anyone can use a pendulum, but you have to be open and relaxed'

## HOW TO ASK YOUR PENDULUM QUESTIONS

Keep the questions simple to get the clearest answers and remember to be specific. Yes and no questions will offer more accurate responses, or 'Show me the direction of . . .'

A meditation practice helps to cultivate a clutter-free mind for exercises like this. If you're distracted, the pendulum could be mistaken and answer one of your stray thoughts instead of the question.

Be mindful when using the pendulum for future predictions because it can be influenced by what you desire, so keep an open mind when trying to tune into the future. In my own experience of using a pendulum to sneak a peek into the future, the answers haven't always been very reliable because emotions and attachments act as a diversion to the truth. I believe that we have a trajectory based on our circumstances and beliefs but your destiny is indefinite because you have free will, which is the power to change your direction in any given way, based on the decisions you make. Your future is your choice and a manifestation of how you respond to the present moment.

### Working with other crystals

You could ask, Is this crystal's energy in harmony with mine? Does this crystal want to work with me? Will this crystal support my friend? Does this crystal need cleansing/charging/reprogramming?

'When working with the pendulum, specific yes or no questions are best'

## Assessing your chakras

You could ask, Show me the direction that the heart chakra (for example) is flowing. The pendulum will respond in a circular movement to indicate the chakra is healthy and open; it will move back and forth to indicate that the chakra is open but the energy is misdirected or being drained; it will move erratically to indicate that the chakra's flow is confused; it will be still if the chakra is closed.

## Checking in with your aura

You could ask, Show me how my aura is today. If the pendulum moves in a large circle, it may mean that you're relaxed; a smaller movement may indicate that you're tired or feel as if you need to protect your energy; if it moves quickly, it may mean that you're energized.

## Finding something that's lost

Hold the pendulum over a map or in places where you think that the lost item may be and ask, Is what I'm looking for here? Wait for the pendulum to respond and try different locations until you find what you're looking for.

These are all suggestions. Inevitably the more you practise with your pendulum, the better you'll understand what its movements mean to *you*.

## What to do when you get an 'I don't know' answer from your pendulum

You've got two options: (a) reframe the question and try again, or (b) trust that sometimes you aren't supposed to know the answer (yet). In that case, put the pendulum away and carry on with your day regardless of what you may have hoped the pendulum would reveal. Sometimes the answer isn't yours to know. It's always your responsibility to create a life that feels aligned with you, regardless of what the pendulum does or doesn't tell you.

## WHEN TO USE YOUR PENDULUM

You can use the pendulum whenever you want to but it's important not to rely on it as the basis for all of your decisions and actions. The pendulum is just an extension of your intuition and what you already know. First and foremost, always trust yourself.

# CRYSTAL HEALING: BODY LAYOUT

**Crystals can facilitate a healing process in the body by harmonizing conflicting energies and realigning the mind, body and spirit. They activate our innate healing powers and remind us that transformation ultimately comes from within. This medicine is available to anyone who's open to receive support.**

Metaphysics recognizes that stress, trauma, unprocessed emotions and stagnant energy can inhibit the body's natural processes, which causes imbalances and can impact on your health. When you feel calm and relaxed, it's so much easier for your body to heal and regenerate efficiently.

This simple layout will help you relax and receive crystal healing.

## You will need

Sage, palo santo or crystal cleansing spray (see page 108)
Four crystals, of your choice

## What to do

- Choose somewhere quiet where you can lie down comfortably, without any distractions. Wear warm layers or use a blanket in case you get cold.

- Stream some calming music and switch your phone to flight mode so that you aren't disturbed. You could also set a timer for twenty–sixty minutes, depending on how long you want to chill out.

- Use sage, palo santo or crystal cleansing spray to bless the area for the ritual.

- Cleanse and programme your crystals – you can do this individually or as a group.

- You will need to lie on your back with your body straight.

- Place the first crystal at the soles of your feet before you lie back. When you're lying down, place the second crystal at the top of your head and hold the remaining crystals, one in each hand. Rest your arms by your sides. The crystals should be positioned to create a diamond shape.

- Take a few gentle, deep breaths and imagine that you're breathing into your heart chakra and, as you exhale, your heart begins to open like the petals of a flower.

- Allow yourself to relax.

- When you feel calm and your thoughts have slowed, send your attention to the crystal at your feet. Visualize it becoming activated and imagine it sending a laser beam of light towards the crystal in your left hand. The beam will activate the crystal (in your left hand) and will continue on to the crystal above your head; the beam will then extend to the crystal in your right hand, back towards the crystal at your feet.

- Visualize yourself within a diamond-shaped circuit of crystalline energy.

- Imagine the crystals' colours radiating and expanding to fill the diamond.

- Spend at least twenty minutes within the crystal layout and imagine yourself absorbing the crystals' energy.

- Be compassionate towards any distractions. It's okay if your thoughts wander from time to time. Allow yourself to be guided back by your breathing or tune into the music.

- Observe any shifts, messages, insights or inspirations that come to you during this time.

- When you're ready, slowly become aware of your surroundings. Gather the crystals in the opposite direction in which you placed them. Disconnect from the energy of each crystal and express gratitude to it as you remove it from the layout.

- Ground yourself: you can do this by stretching, rubbing your hands together, massaging your feet, walking barefoot on grass and/or eating some root vegetables. Drink plenty of water, too.

- Before you carry on with your day, take some time to record your experience.

- Cleanse the crystals after the ritual and keep them close to you for the next twenty-four hours.

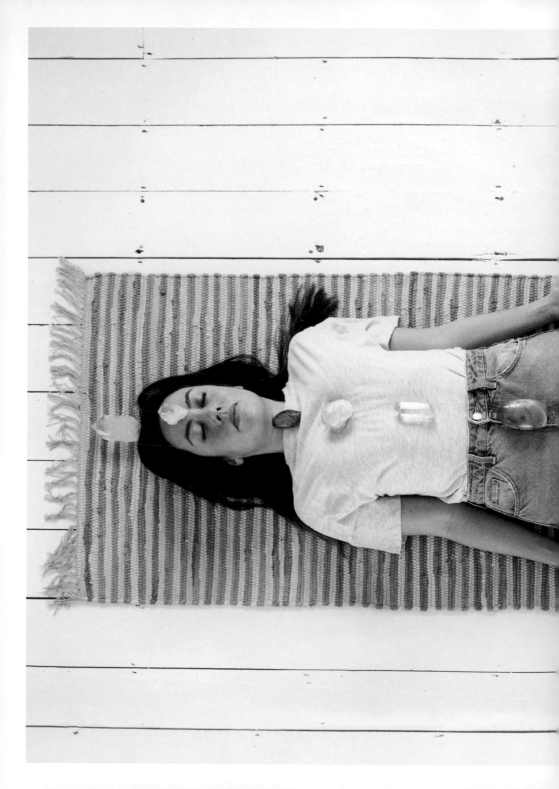

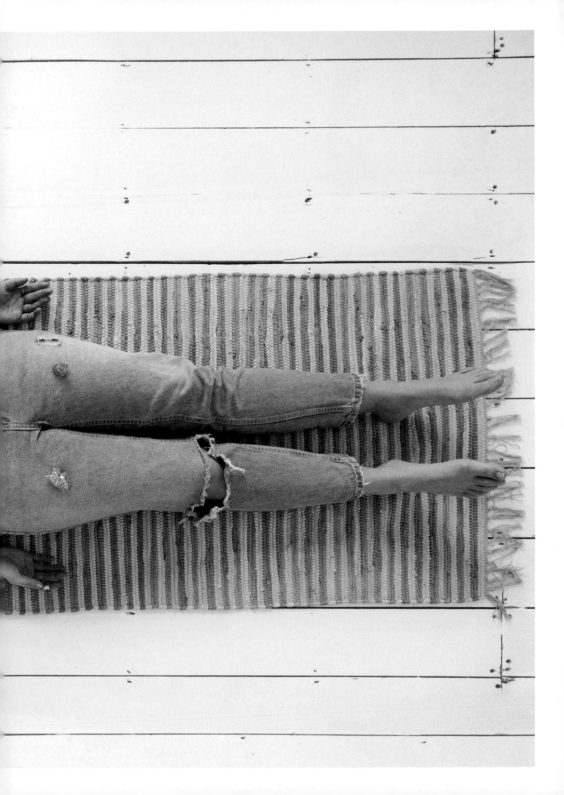

# MASURU EMOTO: THE HEALING POWER OF WATER

**I've been fascinated by the work of Masuru Emoto ever since I came across his work a few years ago. Masuru Emoto is renowned for his studies in the consciousness of water and his breathtaking water-crystal photography. For many years he's examined the healing power of water by exploring how various influences can affect its structure. His hypothesis was that when water's frozen, the ice crystals would reveal its *state*.**

Emoto and his team investigated water from different sources and the impact on it of exposing it to a range of situations. They devised a technique to photograph the frozen water and record how water reacted to different 'experiences'. In *The Healing Power of Water*, Emoto wrote,

> As water freezes, its molecules systematically connect and form the nucleons of a crystal; it becomes stable when it has the structure of a hexagon. This is a natural course of the procedure. However, if unnatural information is forced upon it, it's not able to form a harmonic hexagonal crystal.

Water from natural springs formed stunning crystals with a regular hexagonal structure, whereas water from estuaries and dams struggled to create them. The negative effect of 'chlorine-ridden' water was obvious. The team went on to study the emotional effects of water by labelling it with words; some was exposed to kind and loving words, like 'given a soul' and 'thanks', while other water was subjected to derogatory and cruel words. Research was also extended to the effect of music on water: music of various genres was played to water before it was frozen. The results were astounding. You may have guessed that the water which had been exposed to the loving words and harmonious music created stunning crystals, while water shown hostility and heavy metal music struggled to form any.

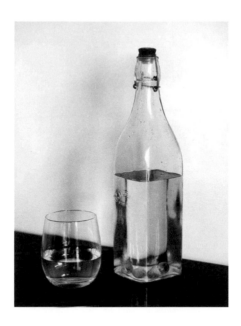

Masuru Emoto's work shows us the hidden properties of water and clearly illustrates that water has a consciousness and demonstrates the impact on it of the environment and thoughts. Consequently, it's not just about water, it's about *us* (and everything else that lives on our planet). The human body is composed of between 55 and 75 per cent water, and so much of our planet (which is 72 per cent water) would be unable to exist without it. What strikes me most about water's ability to form crystals is that we can improve its quality within our bodies through our thoughts, what we choose to surround ourselves with and how we nourish ourselves. Just imagine the crystals you could create within you. We have the potential to reverse the negative impact we're having on our planet by living more consciously, avoiding GMOs (genetically modified organisms), reducing pollution and waste, recycling, saving the rainforest, protecting our water, picking up litter from the beach, saving the bees, being more loving and compassionate in our thoughts and actions . . .

We take water for granted. It's vital for our survival and if we developed a stronger appreciation for it, we could make a difference in so many ways.

# CRYSTALS AND WATER

**When water and crystals are combined, something magical happens. The water becomes activated by the crystal. The crystal's personality (or vibration) is imprinted on the water, which acts as a conduit to transfer the crystal's powers.**

In the same way that Masuru Emoto has shown us that water has a consciousness and is responsive to various influences, this theory (the effect of positive intentions) can be applied when crystals and water are united. I'd love to see the result of water crystals created by infusing the energy of crystals and water.

Remember, not all crystals are water-friendly: some will dissolve in water or rust and others contain mercury or lead, which are toxic. Please check before you experiment with your crystals. If in doubt, leave it out or use an indirect method.

## CRYSTAL ELIXIR

Making an elixir with crystals is one of the easiest and most digestible* ways to soak up some good vibes from the inside out. Sipping crystal-enhanced water throughout the day not only keeps you hydrated but will enhance the transmission of crystal healing. There's a noticeable difference in how water tastes after crystals have been infused in it: I think it tastes cleaner, if that's possible.

### You will need

- 1–3 tumbled stones (of your choice)
- Pen and paper
- Something to infuse your crystal elixir in. I'd recommend a glass Kilner jar but you can use a clean jam jar or jug
- Spring or filtered water
- Drinking glass
- Large bowl (for indirect method)

---

* It's obvious that crystals themselves aren't edible and I wouldn't recommend trying to swallow one to get a dose of vitamin crystal.

## How to create your own crystal elixir

- Tune in to your intention for your elixir: how would you like it to support you? Select one or a few tumbled stones for this purpose. To boost the crystals in your elixir, include a Clear Quartz crystal. Create your own combinations and remember to check which crystals are safe to use in an elixir.

- To sterilize the crystals before use, place them in a saucepan or Pyrex bowl with boiling water. Use a clean spoon to remove the crystal and allow it to cool.

- Begin by cleansing and dedicating your crystals. You can also write your intention or a positive affirmation on a piece of paper and keep it with your elixir while it infuses.

- Place the crystals in a jar and fill with spring or filtered water. Leave the crystals to infuse with the water, either in the sunlight or moonlight. Kilner jars are ideal because they prevent the water from being contaminated during the infusion process while still allowing light to penetrate the elixir.

- *Indirect method.* Fill a clear glass jar with spring or filtered water. Put the water container in a larger glass bowl and place your chosen crystals around it. This way the crystals' energy can infuse the water safely.

- While the elixir is infusing, you can place a small crystal grid around it to magnify the effects (for inspiration, see page 77).

- After at least twelve hours, remove the crystals and transfer the elixir to a drinking glass or water bottle.

- Specific water bottles are available with integrated gemstone pods that make drinking crystal elixirs convenient and stylish. Check out VitaJuwel glass water bottles for more information.

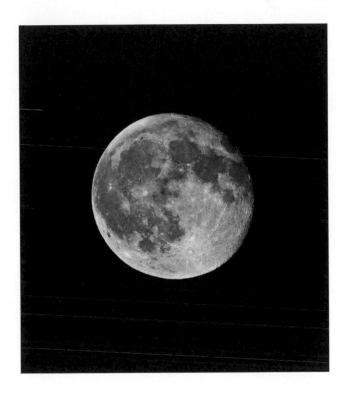

# CRYSTALS AND THE MOON

Not a full moon goes by without someone on social media kindly reminding us to cleanse and charge our crystals. The reason is simple: the full moon has the power to amplify energy and intentions. The moon and crystals are natural guides and healers; together they become a united force of supercharged medicine.

It takes the moon about 27.32 days to orbit the earth and return to its starting position. Its gravitational pull (combined with the sun) is known to influence the ocean's tides, and as we're composed of up to 75 per cent water, this can be seen as an indication of why we feel as we do around the time of the full moon. When the moon is at its fullest, it can turn up the volume to your intuition. I know a lot of people who say they can tell that it's a full moon without even looking up at the night sky because they seem to be more emotionally sensitive, more intuitive, more empathic, find it harder to sleep at night, more inclined to share their opinion or have an argument/misunderstanding, and a greater awareness of things coming to fruition around this time.

The moon also represents the divine feminine (which is in all of us, women and men) and, according to astrology, she rules emotions, intuition, the subconscious, mother, nurturing, food, home, cycles and ancestral roots. With all of this said, I find it hard to believe that it's just a coincidence that a woman's menstrual cycle is on average twenty-eight days and that some women (whose cycle isn't inhibited by contraception and other medications) are in sync with the moon, whether it be the full or new moon.

We, like the moon, are cyclical creatures. Despite constant striving, we aren't linear. Very rarely is there a direct path to happiness and success (whatever form that takes for you). So much happens in the spaces between. Life gets in the way and it can seem as if you're catapulted off course. She – the moon – is there to remind us to go with the flow: in the same way that she has cycles, so do we, and when we embrace them, instead of overriding our intuition, our authenticity has a chance to shine through.

If you tracked your energy levels/moods every day, over time you'd see a pattern emerge. You could also make note of what crystals you're drawn to at different times. Understanding when you're most likely to feel energized or tired can be radically life-changing. It can offer you the opportunity to adjust your lifestyle and schedule accordingly, guiding you to establish positive boundaries and avoid/reduce situations that trigger stress and anxiety, so that you can flow with your own natural rhythm instead of swimming against the tide.

Of course, crystals aren't just for when the full moon aligns: they can help you get to know yourself throughout each phase and support you in harnessing the opportunities that are being illuminated.

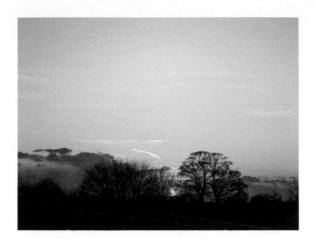

## NEW MOON RITUAL

The new moon is when the moon appears to be dark in the sky. This is because the moon is positioned between the sun and the earth. The side that faces us doesn't receive direct sunlight so the moon isn't visible to us from the earth. This signifies the first phase of the moon; while some consider the new moon to be when it's in total darkness, it can also be thought of as when we see the first glimmer of light on its face. New moons are the ideal time to sow the seeds of new intention. Envisage what you'd like to manifest and begin new projects. What are you ready to begin? What new opportunities are you open to inviting into your life?

Choose a crystal that you'd like to work with for the next moon cycle. This could be intuitively selected or an energy that you know you'd like to support you at this time. Energy flows where intention goes – the sooner that you get crystal clear with your intentions, the sooner you can start attracting more of the good stuff.

### You will need

One crystal* of your choice

Four Quartz points*

Crystal wand or Quartz point to activate the grid

Magazines

Scissors

Glue

Cardboard or canvas

* Cleanse and programme crystals before the ritual (see pages 27 and 38).

## What to do

- Follow the How to Meditate with Crystals meditation (see page 64) to tune in. Think about what you'd like to manifest with the support of your crystal and this new moon. This could be a feeling, an experience, an opportunity, healing, or something you'd like to come into your possession. To harness this moon's powers, you could research the zodiac sign it aligns with for more insight into its magic.

- Write your intention on the canvas/cardboard, then begin cutting out words or images from the magazines that resonate and represent what you'd like to manifest. Give yourself permission to dream big.

- Mindfully arrange and stick your cut-outs on to your canvas/cardboard to create a vision board. Use these words and images to express yourself. Be as creative as you like.

- Look out for any themes from your subconscious that are revealed through your vision board. Take some time to reflect, and record any insights or inspirations that you found from doing this ritual.

- Find somewhere that you can set up your crystal grid and vision board where it can be left undisturbed.

- Lay your vision board flat. Place the main crystal at the centre or in front of it, and lay the Quartz points around the crystal in the directions of north, east, south and west.

- Use the crystal wand or Quartz point to activate the crystal grid (see page 77).

- Say, 'I surrender to the outcome and I'm open to this or something better, thank you.' Leave the crystal grid on your vision board for at least twelve hours or until the next full moon (or longer).

## WAXING MOON RITUAL

Following the new moon, its light grows until the moon becomes full again. When you can see exactly half the moon illuminated while the other half is shadowed, this phase is ideal for taking inspired action towards your intentions. Less procrastination, more manifestation. It's time to take action. You can harness this phase of the moon to support change and transformation. It'll encourage you to move forward so that you can accomplish your passion projects. Consider: what could you do this week that will support you in achieving your dreams? You might craft a fresh CV so that you can apply for a new job, book a course that will give you the skills to do something that inspires you, make your meditation practice non-negotiable, expand your tribe and connect with people you admire.

Ideal crystals to work with at this time include: Citrine, Pyrite, Garnet, Ruby, Rutilated Quartz, Calcite, Sunstone.

### What to do

- Meditate with a crystal (see page 64) and visualize your aspirations coming to fruition. Our beliefs create our reality and visualizations can support us to have more self-trust and confidence.

- Schedule time in your agenda to dedicate to your passion project. If it's scheduled you limit the chance of being sidetracked because you've made a vital commitment to yourself. Ask someone to be your accountability partner so that you've got someone to support you.

- Break your goal into sizeable tasks: focus on what you can do today, this week or next month, before anything else. You'll feel less overwhelmed and more confident if the steps are more realistic and achievable.

- Make a crystal elixir (see page 96) for motivation.

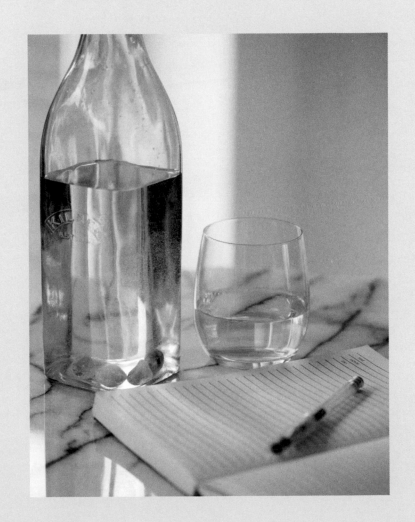

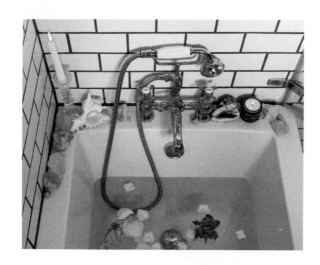

## FULL MOON: BATH RITUAL

When the moon is at its fullest, the earth is positioned between the moon and the sun. The reflection of the sun illuminates the moon, which is why it appears bigger and brighter. The full moon is oh-so-mesmerizing for many of us and has been since the beginning of time. It's believed to be a potent moon phase that amplifies energy. 'Feeling feelings' is a phrase that is often used around this time because, like the moon, everything seems bigger and more intense. This can be a time when hidden truths are brought to the surface and truth bombs are flying around, which can be both liberating and overwhelming. When the moon is at her fullest, it's an invitation to be bold with your aspirations: it invites you to step out of your comfort zone and start making steps towards positive change. It's a nudge to celebrate your achievements, express gratitude and enjoy being more sensual.

### You will need

Crystals* (suggestions: Moonstone, Rose Quartz, Larimar, Aquamarine and Kunzite)

Seashells

Flowers, fresh or dried

Dead Sea salt (alternatively, use Himalayan salt or Epsom salts)

Candles

Muslin drawstring bag (optional)

## What to do

- Place seashells around the bath and light some candles.

- You can either place the crystals and flowers loosely in the bath or in a muslin drawstring bag to keep them all together. Remember that not all crystals are compatible with water: you can place the crystals around the outer edges of the bath or create a crystal grid around the bath. As you place each flower or petal in the water, think of or name aloud something you are grateful for.

- Add two handfuls of natural salt to the bath.

- Fill the bath with water, ensuring that it's a comfortable temperature and depth.

- Relax and soak in the bath for as long as you like.

- When you've finished in the bath, instead of rushing to get out, remove the crystals, pull the plug and remain in the bath until all of the water has drained away. Visualize any unwanted energy being drawn away from you.

If you don't have a bath you could do this ritual either with a footbath or decorate your shower with flowers, crystals and seashells.

# 'A time when hidden truths are brought to the surface and truth bombs are flying around, which can be both liberating and overwhelming'

* Cleanse and programme crystals before this ritual (see pages 27 and 38).

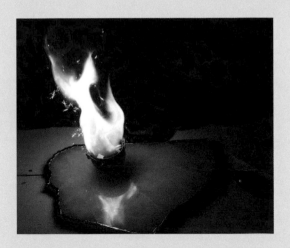

## WANING MOON RITUAL

In the waning moon phase the sunlight has a less visible effect on the moon and it becomes partially shadowed as it moves towards the new moon again. This phase is ideal for letting go of the past, casting spells for protection and banishing, having a closet cleanse and detoxing. It's the time of the moon when you're invited to forgive and release the old to make way for the new. Think of it as an opportunity to perform a ritual that says goodbye to a toxic relationship or to unburden yourself of responsibilities that are way past their use-by date so that you have more time and energy to do the things you *really* want to do. This also includes committing to rewiring old programming that tricks you into thinking you're 'not good enough' for something better. Because you most definitely are.

### What to do

- Meditate (see page 64) with Clear Quartz, Smoky Quartz, Black Obsidian, Snowflake Obsidian, Black Tourmaline, Labradorite or Malachite.

- Consider: what are you ready to let go of so that you can make space to feel more fulfilled? Take some time to record your answers to this question.

- Write a list of habits, thought processes, attachments and situations that you're ready to release.

- Burn (somewhere safe) or bury the list to set yourself free from the attachment.

- Spritz yourself with the crystal cleansing spray or have a crystal bath to finish the ritual.

## WANING MOON: DETOXIFYING SALT SCRUB

Letting go, saying no, setting clear boundaries, sprinkled with love and forgiveness, is what the waning moon is all about. I know that this isn't always the easiest thing to put into practice. After you've done the waning moon ritual, I'd recommend crafting the salt scrub for yourself (maybe make enough for a friend who needs it too).

Our skin is the biggest organ of the body and is always grateful for TLC. It's also the contact point to the aura, which is constantly processing the energies around you and can absorb some undesirable vibes from your day – especially if it's been particularly stressful.

You can use this scrub whenever you want to cleanse and reinvigorate your energy, as an alternative to smudging with sage or palo santo (see page 27). I often use it as a self-care ritual: I visualize shedding the old and revealing the new as I gently massage the salt into my skin. It makes it feel so soft, while the Smoky Quartz and essential oils instantly dissipate any overwhelming feeling and anxiety, leaving me calm and reset.

### Ingredients

200g coconut oil

120g fine Himalayan pink salt

Essential oils: basil, bergamot and geranium

Smoky Quartz tumbled stone

### What to do

- Blend the coconut oil and salt together in a bowl. If you live somewhere cold, warm the coconut oil slightly to soften before adding the salt – this will make it easier to blend.

- Add ten–fifteen drops of your essential oils (I'd suggest five drops of each essential oil, more or less, depending on your desired strength) to the mix and stir it all together.

- Put your Smoky Quartz into a jar and transfer the salt scrub blend so that it can infuse with the crystal. Make sure that the jar has a tight-fitting lid and place it in sunlight or moonlight for twelve hours to activate the scrub.

- Apply the scrub to damp skin while you're in the bath or shower. Be careful because it can make surfaces slippery. Spend some time relaxing in the bath or shower after you've applied the scrub and rinse away your worries.

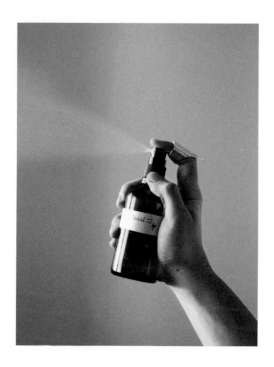

# CRYSTAL CLEANSING SPRAY

It isn't always convenient to burn sage or palo santo to cleanse your crystals, especially when there are fire alarms that love to wake up the neighbourhood, and flatmates who have an aversion to smoke. This is a quick-fix on-the-go crystal cleansing spray that's easy to make and even easier to use. It will cleanse and neutralize any stagnant and unwanted energy with just a few light spritzes. I love how fresh it smells: it's an instant pick-me-up for crystals, home, workspace and humans alike. You can use it any time and (almost) anywhere. Avoid direct contact with electrical items and anything else that isn't liquid-friendly.

## You will need

Spring or filtered water

Clear Quartz or Citrine*

Witch hazel

Essential oils: sage, rosemary, palma rosa

100ml glass bottle with atomizer

I prefer glass bottles as they reduce the use of plastic as well as protecting the spray from heat, oxygen and moisture that can reduce its shelf life. Coloured glass (amber or cobalt blue) is also recommended when using essential oils to protect them from sunlight, which may cause them to evaporate.

## How to make your crystal cleansing spray

- Place the crystal in a glass jug or jar and fill with spring or filtered water. Kilner jars are good because they prevent the water from being contaminated during the infusion process, while still allowing light to penetrate the water.

- Place jar in sunlight or moonlight for twelve hours to activate the water. *To supercharge this spray, make this water on a full moon.*

- While the crystals and water infuse, you can place a small crystal grid around the jar (for inspiration, see page 77) – try Selenite wands or Quartz points, because they're both known for their cleansing and uplifting powers, or whatever crystals you'd like to add some extra energy to the party.

- Three-quarters fill the glass bottle with crystal-infused water. Add fifteen–twenty drops of your essential oils (for example, five drops sage, five drops rosemary and five drops palma rosa), then cover the opening of the bottle and shake to disperse the oils in the water. Fill the rest of the bottle with witch hazel and shake to mix all of the ingredients together.

- Always shake the bottle before use.

- Hold the bottle at least six inches away and use the spray lightly to mist your crystals, meditation area, yoga mat, bedroom, your aura . . . wherever you want to freshen up the vibes.

* Cleanse and programme the crystal before use (see pages 27 and 38).

# CHAPTER THREE

# CRYSTAL GUIDE

Nothing has taught me more about crystals than going through life with them at my side. The messages that I share within these pages are based on experience and intuition, including some interesting crystal lore and practices I've learnt from my teachers (and the crystals) along the way. My intention is to help you use crystals as guides to viewing your life with a fresh perspective, and perhaps uncover some inner wisdom.

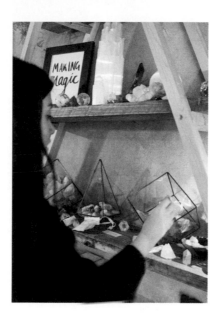

These messages aren't set in stone: over time you will develop your own explanation and meaning for each crystal. A crystal's first task is to switch on your intuition because it's open to interpretation. This is a starting point for you to dive into *your* subconscious and to see how you think and feel. For example, how does a particular crystal make you feel? What was your intention when choosing that one? To what challenges or energies are you opening up? What shifts did you notice after connecting with your crystal?

When you spend time with each stone you'll get to know their personality from the way they make you feel, and learn more about those times when you feel drawn to keep certain crystals close by. I like to think of it as dating your crystals. Just like Tinder dates, crystals have personalities that go way beyond the profile picture. Before you've played out the relationship in your head, go on a few dates with your crystal. Keep the crystal's biography in mind and the reason that you initially chose it: take the crystal out with you and be open to what happens in your day. What happens in your day that reminds you of the crystal and how does the situation play out? Does the crystal inspire you to react differently? For example, say you've chosen Moonstone (see page 202) because you want to start flexing your intuition muscle and you've also noticed that you're feeling burnt out: where in your day could you make time to meditate or delegate so that you could focus on just one thing? Could you give yourself a digital curfew so that you have time to unwind before you go to bed? Where can you invite more flow and space into your day? Use crystals as a reminder of your intention.

**The most powerful meanings of crystals are the ones that you discover yourself.**

# AMAZONITE

## New beginnings, courage, truth, confidence

Amazonite is known as a stone of truth and courage because it invites you to step into your natural talents. This crystal revives your sense of purpose and illuminates your innate superpowers. Amazonite reminds you that there's more to life than working a nine-to-five job that may be chipping away at your soul. Instead of feeling trapped by your current situation, align yourself with projects or a job that excites and inspires you, with a team or tribe that gets you. Amazonite helps you connect with your own mission statement so that you can get rooted in your life purpose. This may involve you in stepping out of the hustle and becoming the CEO of yourself, doing what you love. Are you ready to start saying yes to your ideals so they can become reality?

Use this crystal to focus on dedicating your time and energy to nurturing projects close to your heart. It can help to create clear boundaries. Being busy and overwhelmed is an outdated trophy of success: have this crystal around to remind you that balancing your work, rest and play time will allow everything to flow and keep your mind clear.

Its light-hearted energy can help to relieve any pressure you may be feeling so that you can get over your fear of failure, giving your confidence a boost. It's an ideal talisman when going for an interview or starting a new job, business or venture.

You've got this.

*Venture outside your comfort zone. The rewards are worth it*

| | |
|---|---|
| **PHYSICAL HEALING:** | **Calms the nervous system and supports recovery from illness, trauma and injury; also helps with throat issues and chest problems** |
| **CHAKRA:** | **Heart and throat** |
| **SOURCE:** | **Brazil, Ethiopia, India, Madagascar, Namibia, Russia and USA** |

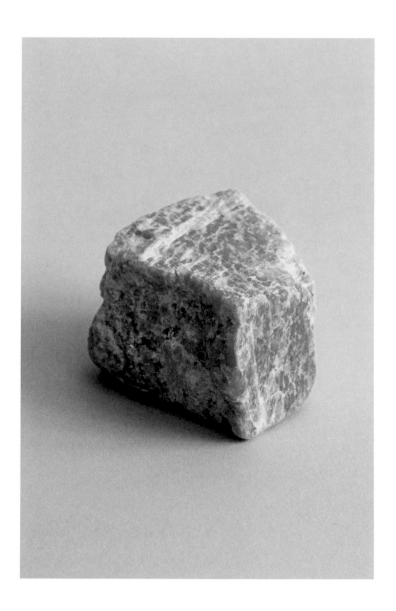

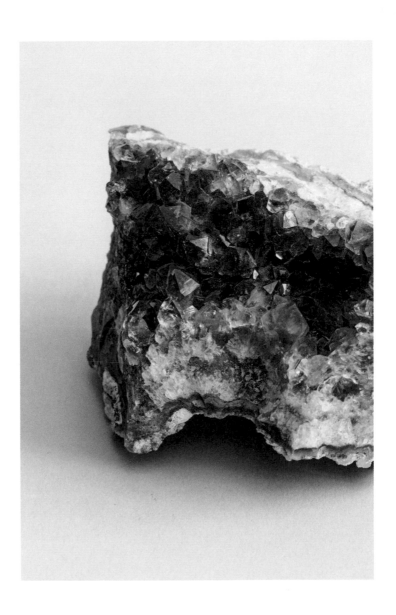

# AMETHYST

## Meditation, calm, sobriety, addictions, sleep

Amethyst is an ultra-calming crystal that can untangle your overactive thoughts so that you have a better view of what's really happening, right here, right now. This one's for the over-thinkers, drama queens and hotheads. Because all of that excessive thinking (a.k.a. obsession) is leading you down a road that leads to Anxietyville. Slow down. Then slow down some more. It's our limiting thought processes that keep us in this spin-cycle, and the only way to change it is to explore new ways of thinking.

Amethyst is said to be a stone of spiritual awakening and I totally get that: when I was at the height of my anxiety and depression I was drawn to it all the time. I'd be so busy overanalysing even the smallest aspects of my day that I'd end up self-sabotaging: I cared too much what other people thought about me, and not enough about me, myself and I. Looking for inner peace? It starts with listening to what you need and taking action towards the things you really want to be doing. This is where your transformation begins.

This stone is well known for helping with stress, anxiety, overwhelming feelings, sleep disorders, overcoming addictions and obsessive thinking.

Instead of numbing life's stresses with alcohol, junk food, social media or online shopping, get curious and spend some down time with this 'stone of sobriety'. Use Amethyst to support a detox or 'dry' January.

*Slow down – your overactive mind is leading you astray. It's time to stop seeking answers and start listening to your intuition*

| PHYSICAL HEALING: | Helps relieve headaches and migraines; lie with a piece of amethyst on your forehead or make a healing crystal elixir (see page 96) |
|---|---|
| CHAKRA: | Third eye |
| SOURCE: | Argentina, Bolivia, Brazil, Canada, Russia, Siberia, South Korea, Sri Lanka, Uruguay and USA |

# AMETRINE (BOLIVIANITE)

## Confidence, boundaries, self-acceptance, balance

Ametrine is a natural fusion of Amethyst and Citrine. Its calming energies (from Amethyst) gently awaken your sense of personal power (represented by Citrine). This crystal illuminates where you're focusing your energy and where you might have some energetic leaks, like other people's demands on your time, leaving you too tired to focus on your own business.

Codependency is a theme with this crystal: are you letting someone overpower your choices or needs? Are you burning yourself out in the hope of gaining external validation? Are you the one who pretends they're laidback and happy to go with the flow when you're just avoiding taking responsibility for your own decisions? Are you saying yes to everyone else's needs and putting yourself at the back of the queue?

If someone asks you to do something or your phone pings with a message, and your body feels heavy with the knot of anxiety in your stomach, it's time to start practising the magic word *No*. Saying no can be the hardest thing to do but Ametrine is there to support you. When you take the opportunity to step back and recharge, so that you can be true to yourself, you'll have more to give.

Ametrine can stabilize your emotions and guide you to become more aware of your triggers so that you can learn how to navigate your way around them. It's a supportive stone when it comes to body positivity, helping to create empowering habits, self-acceptance, overcoming addictions, and teaches us that food is our friend, not the enemy. Keep close to you when you're having therapy or exploring positive lifestyle changes. See also Amethyst (page 117) and Citrine (page 154).

*You have the answers – trust your intuition and take action towards what you need*

| | |
|---|---|
| **PHYSICAL HEALING:** | **Helps relieve headaches and migraines** |
| **CHAKRA:** | **Solar plexus and third eye** |
| **SOURCE:** | **Bolivia and Brazil** |

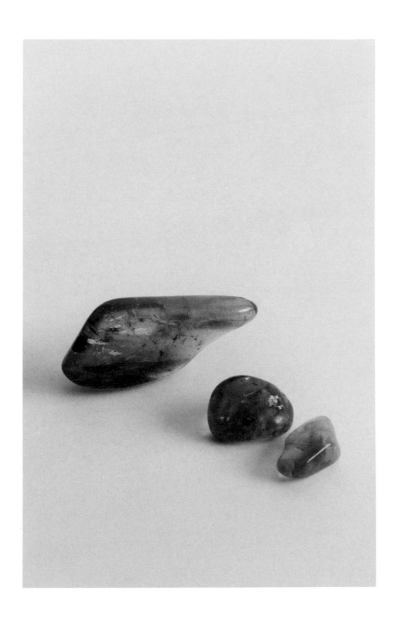

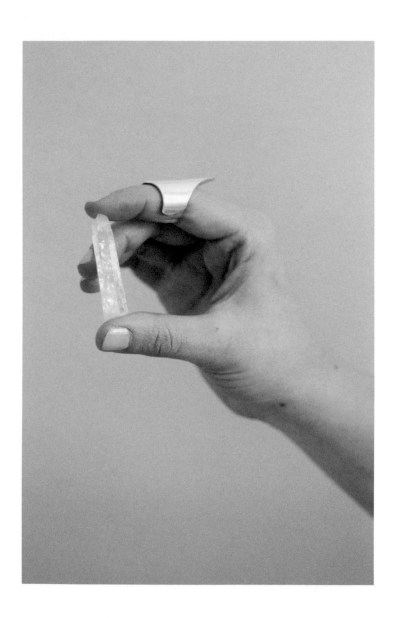

# ANGEL AURA

## Angels, freedom, inspiration, synchronicity

Angel Aura is an enhanced crystal, created through a process of electrostatically fusing Quartz with platinum, silver and gold. This gives the crystal a unique iridescent sheen that makes it look like it's been glittered up for a festival. It's called Angel Aura because of its resemblance to the gossamer wings of angels, and it's said to help you access the angelic realms.

The rainbow of colours that shimmers across the surface of this crystal will bring an uplifting and playful energy to any situation. If you're yearning to dance around in a field at the weekend with your crew, but instead you're stuck at your desk with FOMO (fear of missing out), get some Angel Aura into your life. It will help balance your chakras, stimulating your energetic system and dissolving any energy blockages. Festival vibes, without the hangover.

You can meditate with Angel Aura to open your heart and mind to angels. These benevolent beings will always support you when you ask for their guidance and assistance. Angel Aura is a reminder to trust in the process, that everything is as it's meant to be, so that you feel you're in sync with the universe because everything's going to be more than okay.

When you connect with Angel Aura, don't be surprised if you start noticing synchronicities around you, such as seeing angelic numbers, like 111 or 222, on either a clock or a shopping receipt. Other signs are white feathers, white butterflies and any other angelic representations that resonate with you. These help you to know your angels are with you and that you're always loved and supported.

*Synchronicities are love notes from the universe, showing that you're moving in the right direction*

| PHYSICAL HEALING: | Releases stress, tensions and anxiety stored in your body |
|---|---|
| CHAKRA: | Crown |
| SOURCE: | Man-made |

# APATITE

## Past lives, animal conservation, community, self-awareness

Apatite comes in different colours and formations. Its name in Greek means 'to deceive' because it was often mistaken for other minerals. It's also a phosphate found in teeth and bones, as well as the tusks, horns and antlers of animals. Yes, we've got crystals hidden in our teeth and bones.

Apatite calls you to be part of a community, to bring the planet into love and harmony, protecting everyone and everything.

It will activate your intuition. Your subconscious holds so much juicy wisdom that can help you realize repeated patterns that are manifesting in your current situation, like attracting emotionally unavailable lovers or jobs where you're undervalued. Realizing the cycle is the catalyst to *breaking* it. You're here to evolve. Don't give yourself a hard time for getting things wrong or misjudging people. It's okay to make mistakes because that's how you learn.

This is a stone of empowerment that encourages you to make peace with the past and present so you can build a brighter future. It'll help you break negative cycles of self-sabotage. Understanding how you're rooted in the past will help you move forward.

Live the process. This is how we heal and grow.

*Dear Past, thank you for the lessons. Dear Future, let's do this differently*

| | |
|---|---|
| **PHYSICAL HEALING:** | **Can be used to remedy headaches and is said to enhance eyesight, support broken bones and strengthen teeth** |
| **CHAKRA:** | **Third eye and throat** |
| **SOURCE:** | **Canada and Russia** |

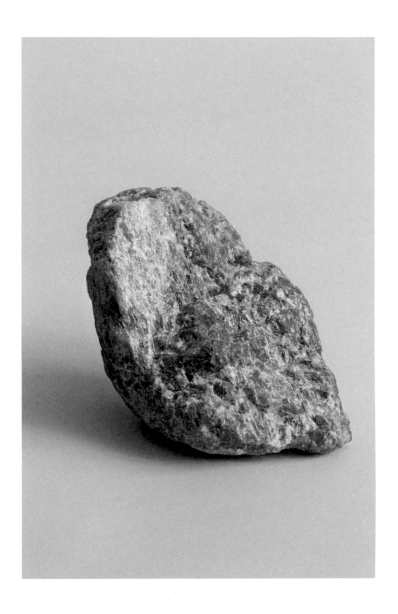

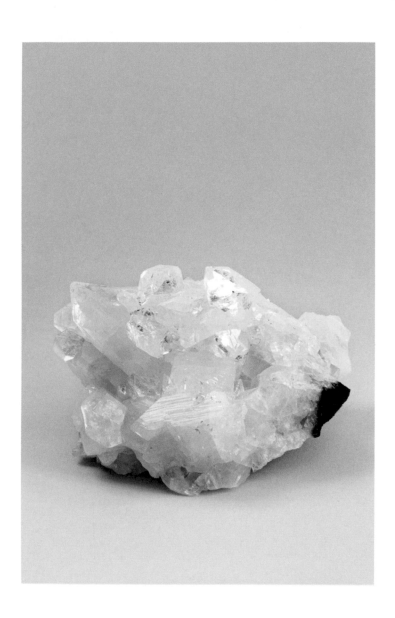

# APOPHYLLITE

## Clarity, new beginnings, Reiki, spiritual awakening

Apophyllite is an uplifting crystal that has an affinity with Reiki and other spiritual realms. It helps you to attune to the universal frequencies of love and light by activating your crown chakra so that you can connect with your authenticity.

Apophyllite loves to create space for you to embrace your feelings and blow away the cobwebs (a.k.a. the burden of all of the things you think you 'should' be doing/feeling/saying, or attachments that you need to let go). If your life is resembling a pity party for one, stop making excuses and start doing the things that support you: it's the only way that things will change.

*Self-care isn't selfish.* Ask for support; team up with a mentor or life coach; explore different avenues of personal development; sign up to a workshop or course that inspires you; have a healing session or tarot reading; go to a sound bath; practise meditation; call a friend to talk things out. Basically, do whatever ignites a spark in you because that's what you need. If you don't know what that is, get curious – try something new and see where it takes you. It's about getting out of your own way so that you can start flowing with life again.

When it comes to new beginnings in your love life, Apophyllite will help you check out of Heartbreak Hotel and lean into the fact that history doesn't have to repeat itself, as long as you've learnt the lessons you needed to from the last relationship. If you're in a long-term relationship, Apophyllite will create space for you to express yourself honestly and openly, without playing the blame game. It's all about taking responsibility for your own actions and reactions so that you can move forward.

This crystal is most commonly clear, white or grey, although it can also be green. Green Apophyllite has the same properties as above, while also resonating with nature and earth spirits. Work with the green crystal to connect with the consciousness of plants, trees, rocks and animals.

*Overcome your limitations and get creative with what you can do now*

PHYSICAL HEALING: **Releases stress, tensions and anxiety stored in your body**

CHAKRA: **Crown and third eye**

SOURCE: **Brazil, Canada, Germany, Greenland, India and Italy**

# AQUAMARINE

## Loyalty, joy, calm, emotional healing

Aquamarine is a youthful crystal that brings joy and happiness. It's the kind of crystal that makes you feel like a Care Bear and want to send out love beams to everyone.

This is the crystal that you want at your side when clear and honest communication is a must. Speaking from the heart and remembering to listen to what the other person has to say will open doors that were closed before. It's important to side-step what you *think* you're entitled to, or what's fair, and be open to negotiation so that the outcome benefits the highest good of all. Sometimes things don't work out as you'd anticipated but it's ultimately leading you in a better direction. It's all part of a bigger picture and you'll probably look back ten years from now grateful that things worked out this way.

Aquamarine also helps illuminate emotional patterns, bringing things to the surface, so they can be acknowledged and healed. It can guide you to reprogramme outdated thought processes and attachments; it's a great support crystal if you're having therapy or counselling. When suffering from grief, Aquamarine is there to help you to let go so that you can start moving forward, while still feeling the special bond with the spirit and memories of your loved one.

The soothing energies of Aquamarine can calm highly strung, emotionally sensitive and angry people, preventing mood swings, tantrums and meltdowns, so it's great for toddlers, teenagers, hotheads and drama queens. It's definitely for anyone who gets road rage, too. Aquamarine's medicine is: stop trying to rush, manipulate or control the outcome and embrace what's happening right now.

Aquamarine has an affinity with the element of water and is associated with mermaids and protecting sailors on their voyages. When you're travelling overseas, it can save you from delays or complications.

*Everything is aligned*

| | |
|---|---|
| **PHYSICAL HEALING:** | **Believed to soothe the throat and remedy inflammatory diseases** |
| **CHAKRA:** | **Throat and heart** |
| **SOURCE:** | **Afghanistan, Africa, Australia, Brazil, Kenya, Pakistan, Sri Lanka, Tanzania and USA** |

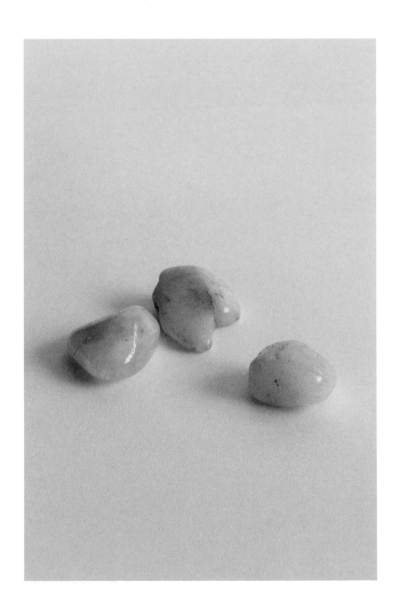

AQUAMARINE

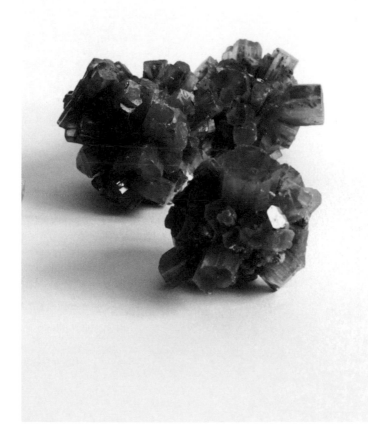

ARAGONITE

# ARAGONITE

## Grounding, anxiety, sleep, new ventures

Aragonite resembles a star cluster; its unusual formations make it look as if it's from outer space. It's said to have the power to harmonize stress on the planet due to construction, mining and fracking, even without direct contact.

This mineral is known as an 'earth healer', and when you connect with it you can sense a deep energy rising up through the earth to support you. It may well inspire you to want to protect the planet and wildlife, or at least to up your recycling game.

Aragonite reminds us that we're all interconnected. We only have one planet to call home, so it's vital we all play our part in preserving and protecting what we have.

With this strong earthy connection, Aragonite will bring a stable and balancing energy to any situation. If you're going through big (sometimes unexpected) changes in your life, keep this mighty mineral close by to help reduce any anxiety you may be feeling. Change is inevitable: it's natural to experience growing pains that lead to you asking *all* the big questions: What's my life purpose? Do I save for a mortgage or go travelling? Do I want children? Shall I relocate overseas? Is this relationship for ever? Whatever *your* big question, take some time to feel into what's true for you before making any drastic decisions. Talk it out with a friend if you need to.

Sleeping with the stone under your pillow can bring you a restful night's sleep, while keeping it close during the day may make you feel more centred and less anxious.

Due to its cluster formation, Aragonite channels energy in different directions and can bring harmony to the collective consciousness, which would be ideal in an office environment, encouraging the kind of teamwork where you're all bouncing ideas together. Its process is swift and can accelerate personal development by clarifying situations. It also boosts concentration and commitment, making it an ally for students, new businesses and when you need to complete a project.

This mineral easily absorbs negative energy so needs to be cleansed regularly (see page 27).

*When you're grounded, you're reminded that you're always supported*

| PHYSICAL HEALING: | Believed to revitalize your energetic system and increase stamina; said to support broken bones in healing |
|---|---|
| CHAKRA: | All |
| SOURCE: | Austria, Czech Republic, England, Greece, Italy, Mexico, Pakistan, Peru and USA |

# AVENTURINE - GREEN

## Prosperity, manifestation, self-worth, receptivity, balance

Green Aventurine is a dynamic crystal, famous for attracting prosperity. Show me the money, I hear you say. The thing is, the likelihood of winning the lottery is pretty small (especially if you don't buy a ticket) but this generous crystal will boost your money-making abilities. To become a clear channel to receive and manifest opportunities, you need to rewire your beliefs around self-worth, or you'll deflect opportunities as soon as they come your way. It's time to start believing you deserve abundance in *all* forms, including love.

Being rich isn't the main objective for everyone but having enough to pay off your debts, a deposit to buy your first home, money for a dream holiday or to invest in a course to kick-start your career can be life-changing. If you've always thought that success, love and wealth happen to other people and you've dubbed yourself the 'unlucky' one, think again. This crystal has come into your life to let you know that everything is possible: you just need to expand your belief system of what you deserve.

Focus on this crystal to cultivate a healthy relationship with money: pay off debts, save for the future, invest, and spend on things that nourish you and others while being grateful for what you receive. Keep a piece of Green Aventurine in your purse and write a little note to go with it, 'Money flows to me', as a reminder that you always have enough and there's always more to come. Do this when you're saving for something special or to alleviate any angst if you're about to make a big investment.

Being abundant means you have more to *give*, and Green Aventurine will balance your energy so you're in sync with giving *and* receiving.

*Abundance is flowing your way*

| | |
|---|---|
| **PHYSICAL HEALING:** | **Believed to enhance a general sense of well-being, support the heart and stimulate cell regeneration when a wound is healing or after medical treatment** |
| **CHAKRA:** | **Heart** |
| **SOURCE:** | **Brazil, India and Russia** |

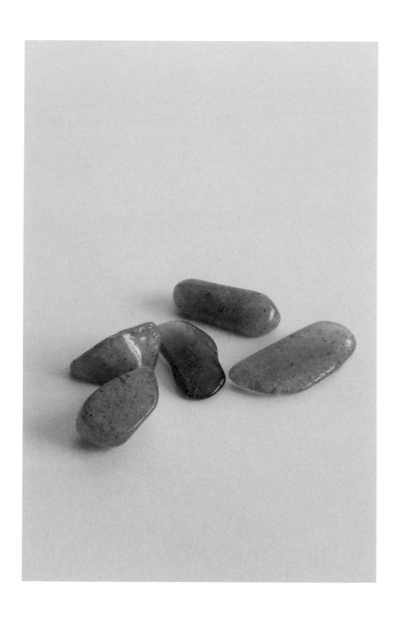

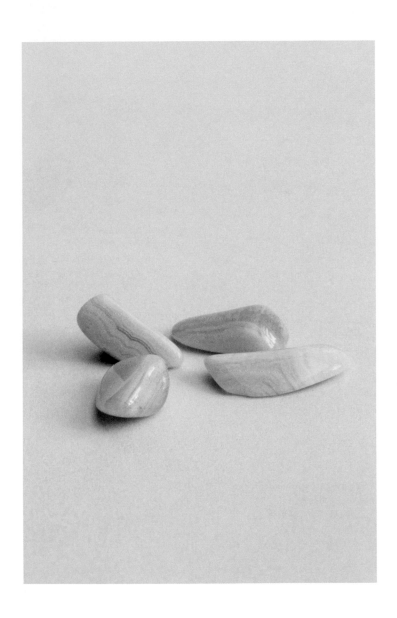

# BLUE LACE AGATE

## Calm, soothing, communication, compassion

If Blue Lace Agate were human, it would be the kind of person who'd run you a relaxing bath after a long day at the office and listen to you moan about what a disaster it's been. It's the friend who makes all of your cares and worries vanish when you're with them because they just get you and you can be real. Blue Lace Agate energy is soft, gentle and reassuring. It's a permission slip to quieten your mind, soothe emotions and calm your nervous system. Holding a piece can help you relax and turn down the volume of any anxiety, making you feel supported.

This crystal is well known for its powers of assisting communication. Choose Blue Lace Agate to help you find your voice and the confidence to express your beliefs and needs. Especially useful when you're public speaking, having an important meeting or a heart-to-heart with your loved one. It's time to stop shying away from using your voice and start speaking your truth. Blue Lace Agate is the one you want on your team to guide you towards forgiveness, bringing disputes or confrontations to a harmonious resolution. It's time to forgive and let go so you've more energy to move forward.

Blue Lace Agate is connected with the angelic realms, so if you ever feel stuck, call on your angels and spirit guides to support you.

Working with this stone will encourage you to speak your intentions and affirmations aloud, giving them more power to manifest.

*I choose words that come from my heart and speak with compassion and clarity*

| | |
|---|---|
| **PHYSICAL HEALING:** | **Believed to reduce inflammation, soothe throat infections and laryngitis** |
| **CHAKRA:** | **Crown, throat and heart** |
| **SOURCE:** | **Romania and South Africa** |

# BRANDBERG AMETHYST

## Spiritual awakening, intuition, healing, new beginnings

Brandberg Amethyst is a naturally occurring fusion of Amethyst, Smoky Quartz and Clear Quartz. It's named after the Brandberg mountain range and sacred site in Namibia where it comes from. Each stone has its own distinctive inclusions of enhydros (water with air bubbles), phantoms (illusion of a crystal within a crystal) and rainbows. You could notice something new about this stone every time you gaze into it – it's mesmerizing.

Brandberg's personality reminds me of the zodiac sign Scorpio. Its deep and mysterious energy will guide you to embrace the shadowy aspects (insecurities, darkest secrets, traumas, fears) of yourself so that you can begin to understand complex emotions: it loves tapping into your subconscious thought processes so that you can realize where you keep tripping yourself up. If you don't examine your life, you're living on autopilot. This crystal is all about rebirth and transformation. Once you've learnt how to integrate your shadow side, you'll rise like the phoenix from the ashes: we need to accept the light *and* the dark to make us feel complete.

This crystal will awaken your inner mystic and take you to another galaxy, given half the chance. Meditate with Brandberg Quartz before doing tarot readings or intuitive work: it can help you tap into a stream of psychic and healing energy. Sleep with it under your pillow to enhance your dreams, making them more vivid and easier to remember – don't forget to write them down in the morning so that you can observe any patterns and decode what they mean.

See also Clear Quartz (page 158), Amethyst (page 117) and Smoky Quartz (page 236).

*Step into the unknown and tap into your potential*

| | |
|---|---|
| **PHYSICAL HEALING:** | **Believed to remedy headaches, migraines, immune deficiencies and chronic fatigue disorders and to provide pain relief** |
| **CHAKRA:** | **Crown, third eye and root** |
| **SOURCE:** | **Namibia** |

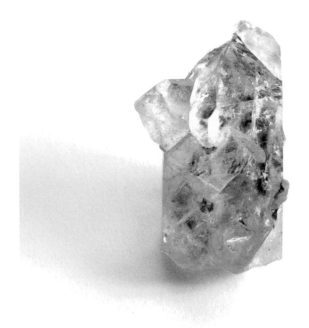

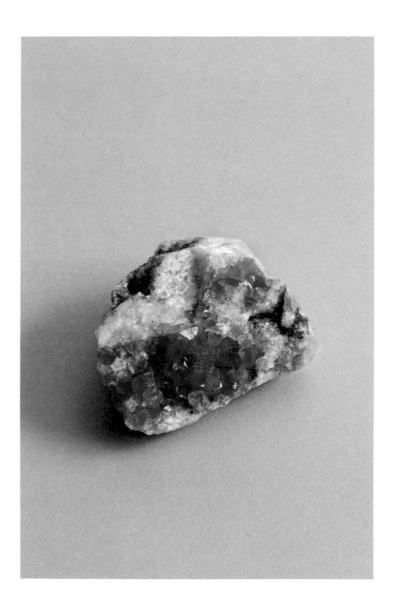

# CALCITE – COBALTO

## (ALSO COBALTOAN CALCITE AND SPHAEROCOBALTITE)

### Transformation, awakening, compassion, optimism, love

Cobalto Calcite is a potent heart activator that will heighten your awareness of how you're expressing love and communicating with others through your words, actions and body language. Is there a disconnection between what you're asking for compared to how you're acting? This is a crystal for reigniting the spark in a long-term relationship when passion has been put on the back burner and routine has led you to take each other for granted. It's time to have some fun together. Looking for a special someone? Maybe you need to stop playing hard to get. Love may be just a right-swipe away, but you need to set up a profile and send Cupid a signal that you're single and ready to mingle. And if your friends want to set you up on a date, why not go for it?

This crystal's unassuming energy has the power to turn up the volume to your sensual side, as well as heal and soothe your heart from past loves.

Think of Cobalto Calcite as the Love Guru: it can inspire you to see and do things in new ways so that you have a better understanding of what you're projecting in relationships, letting go of any fear that history might repeat itself or that you aren't 'good' enough. When you rewrite your love story and remember how amazing you truly are, you'll step fully into love – with or without a relationship.

*Love begins with you*

| | |
|---|---|
| **PHYSICAL HEALING:** | **Believed to boost energy, support recovery from medical procedures and accidents, and reduce pain and heart disorders** |
| **CHAKRA:** | **Heart** |
| **SOURCE:** | **Democratic Republic of Congo, Germany and Morocco** |

# CALCITE - GREEN

## Love, well-being, new beginnings, calming

If a green goddess juice were a crystal, Green Calcite would be the one. This (non-edible) superfood of the crystal realm promotes good health and well-being. It will support you to incorporate rituals and practices into your lifestyle that help you feel more balanced and nourished.

Green Calcite loves to nudge you to show up and see what happens – there's magic to be found in new beginnings and experiences. It's a gentle guide to journey outside your comfort zone so that you can step into your highest potential.

There's a saying, 'Bloom where you're planted' – I think Mary Engelbreit said it first – and Green Calcite is all about helping you make choices that enrich your life and help you grow. You don't have to travel to the other side of the world to 'find yourself': it can happen on your own doorstep. Exploring local neighbourhoods, experimenting with new recipes, reading, signing up for classes, workshops or online courses, finding your tribe: there's so much that can influence how you feel. It can be a combination of what you're eating, the people you're spending time with, your job, how much fresh air you're breathing, the social-media accounts you're following. Maybe it's time for a detox in more ways than one.

Like all calcites, the green version can support your true values, not the ones imposed by other people. Your mission is to feel good, inside and out.

*Just be yourself*

| | |
|---|---|
| **PHYSICAL HEALING:** | **Believed to support the heart and recovery from illness, boost immunity and increase general well-being** |
| **CHAKRA:** | Heart |
| **SOURCE:** | Mexico |

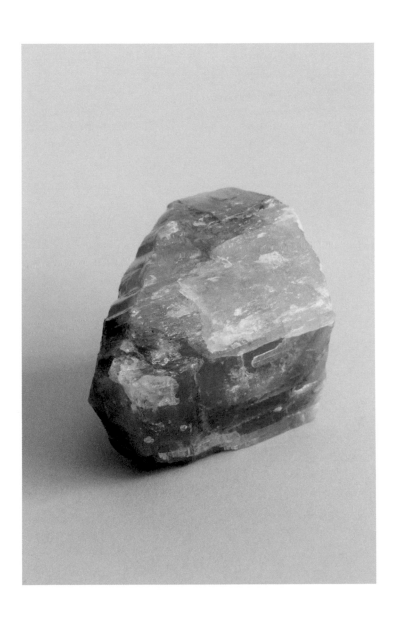

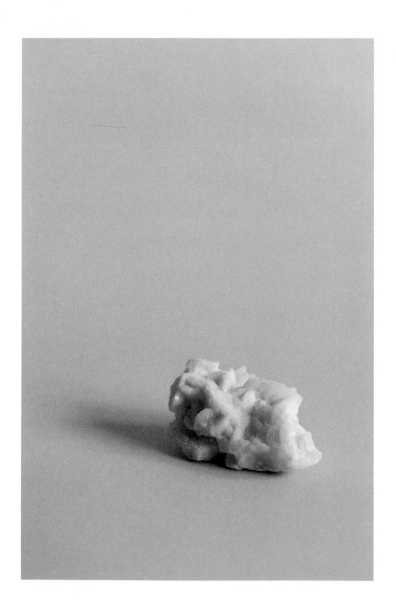

# CALCITE – MANGANO (PINK CALCITE)

## Divine feminine, nurturing, emotional healing, forgiveness

Mangano Calcite is like the mother of the crystal realm. Its energy is kind, gentle, protective and reassuring. It can help you tap into your feminine side and guide you towards living a lifestyle that feels in harmony with your values. When you pick up this crystal, its energy aims to flow straight to your heart. It helps soothe heartache, grief, trauma and unprocessed emotions. As raw as these experiences might feel, they serve to open your heart – not close it. This is a lesson in vulnerability and having to embrace feelings you've been trying to avoid. You've got to feel it to heal it.

Mangano Calcite has an affinity with Reiki energy and supports long-distance healing. It amplifies the sense of empathy – tuning into other people's feelings – even from afar. You don't have to be a Reiki practitioner to make the most of these benefits: give this crystal to someone who needs some love with the intention that when they hold the crystal they feel you giving them a huge hug.

This crystal's nurturing frequency can heal conflict or trauma between parents and children, encouraging harmony and forgiveness. It's also said to help strengthen the bond between mother and baby, especially if there has been a traumatic birth. This is the perfect crystal for a young child to help soothe separation anxiety.*

*You've got to feel it to heal it*

| | |
|---|---|
| **PHYSICAL HEALING:** | **Believed to support recovery after trauma, surgery and heart disorders. Encourages cell regeneration** |
| **CHAKRA:** | **Heart** |
| **SOURCE:** | **Peru** |

* Don't give small stones to babies – place the stones in the room out of reach.

# CALCITE – OPTICAL / CLEAR

## Uplifting, new beginnings, rejuvenation, creativity

Optical Calcite is known as a double-refractive crystal. It has an optical trick in that it gives you double vision when you look directly through it. If you look closely enough, you might even notice rainbows within the crystal. Its energy is cool and refreshing, almost like a breath mint. Hang out with Optical Calcite when you're up against a creative block or just need a little pick-me-up.

When you're too busy, stressed, tired and overwhelmed, it's easy to be fooled into thinking there's only one way of doing things: the hard way. This crystal reminds you there are always two ways – sometimes more – of viewing a situation, always two sides to a story and more than one way of doing things. Bring on those 'aha' moments.

Optical Calcite also encourages you to take a break and get some fresh air. Set yourself free from what you 'should' do and take the weight off your shoulders.

Every moment is an opportunity to start again. What will support you now? It's always easier to find answers when you take time to recharge and try something different.

*When you see things from a different perspective, everything expands*

| | |
|---|---|
| **PHYSICAL HEALING:** | **Believed to help energize and overcome lethargy, boost the metabolism and remedy adrenal fatigue** |
| **CHAKRA:** | **All** |
| **SOURCE:** | **Iceland and Mexico** |

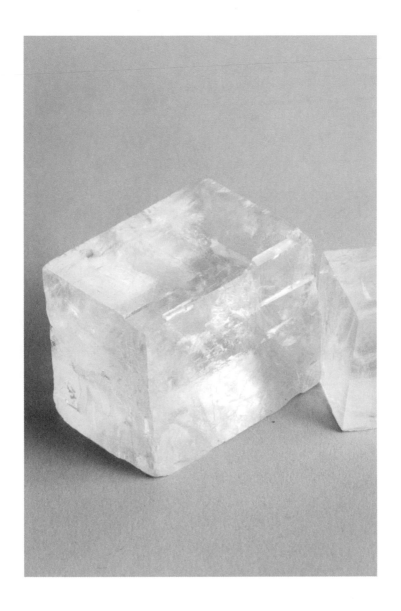

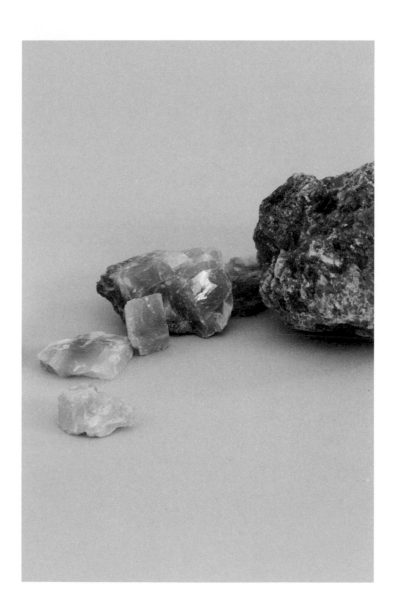

# CALCITE - ORANGE

## Confidence, creativity, passion, fertility

Orange Calcite is like crystallized confidence. It amplifies creative and sexual energy, bringing more passion and excitement your way. This stimulating crystal can empower you to take action.

The things you've been putting off can't wait any longer. It's time to let go of limiting self-beliefs and start nurturing your dreams.

Because Orange Calcite activates your sacral chakra, it's associated with fertility and is said to be an encouraging crystal for pre-conception, low fertility, and to remedy sexual dysfunction.

Wear Orange Calcite to energize you and overcome feelings of lethargy and depression.

*Dream it, real-life it — you have the power!*

| | |
|---|---|
| **PHYSICAL HEALING:** | **Believed to balance hormones and the endocrine system, overcome adrenal fatigue, boost metabolism, support the reproductive system and virility** |
| **CHAKRA:** | **Sacral** |
| **SOURCE:** | **Croatia and Mexico** |

# CARNELIAN

## Action, passion, focus, commitment, confidence

Ready, set, GO! Carnelian is a stone of action and it wants you to know that it's time to start moving. This one's for the commitment-phobes out there. No more excuses. It's energizing and stimulating, like your morning cup of coffee but in crystal form. Keep Carnelian close to you if you need some help staying focused so that you can commit to your goals, especially if you've got a deadline to make.

Stop waiting for life to arrange itself for you and the perfect opportunity to come your way. *You've* gotta make it happen. You need to start making moves and creating opportunities for yourself. Write the proposal you've been procrastinating with, send the email, click 'publish' on the blog post, set up the YouTube channel, put the call out that you're open for business – stand up and get noticed.

Carnelian can support you to take a leap of faith and encourages you to believe in number one. You could think of it as a crystallized dose of confidence. Make a crystal elixir (page 96) with Carnelian so that you can sip decaf motivation throughout the day.

Its fiery personality has the power to ignite passion in all areas of your life, including love, because when you're living in your zone of genius, you lose your old inhibitions and those vibes are electric.

*Feel empowered – the time to take action is now!*

| | |
|---|---|
| **PHYSICAL HEALING:** | Believed to increase stamina, vitality, fertility and virility; keep with you if you suffer from PMT, heavy or painful periods, or you're riding a rollercoaster of hormones and 'hot flushes' from menopause; also said to have detoxifying properties |
| **CHAKRA:** | Solar plexus, sacral and base |
| **SOURCE:** | Brazil, India and Uruguay |

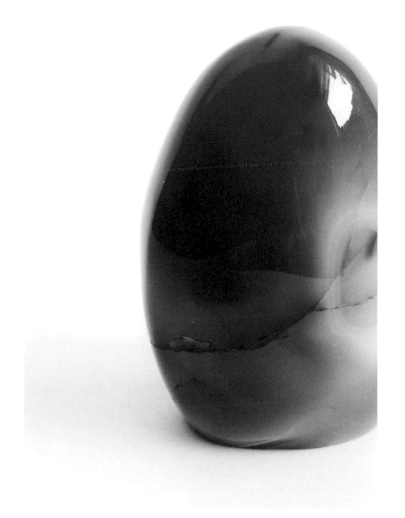

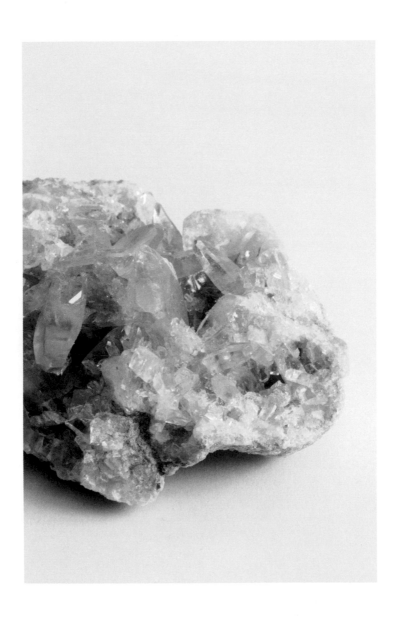

# CELESTITE

## Clarity, honesty, peace, hope and forgiveness

If you were to imagine what it would be like to be in the same room as an angel, with huge soft wings wrapped around you, that's how Celestite can make you feel. Celestite is a direct line to angelic realms, which makes it a calming and uplifting crystal. Its energy is gentle, divine and nurturing. Celestite is the perfect crystal when life takes over and your stress levels are at their peak as it will encourage you to ask for help instead of bearing the burden alone or shouldering outdated responsibilities.

Speak your truth and allow your voice to be heard. Celestite is known to soothe anxiety and bring harmony to situations.

Rise above frustrations and remember that everything happens for a reason. When your overactive mind is leading you astray, practise mindfulness: take a break to meditate somewhere quiet and spend a few minutes to check in and just focus on your breathing, or chill out with a cup of tea (minus scrolling on your phone). It's okay to take a break, especially when you need it.

Meditating with this stone may activate higher states of consciousness. This high-frequency crystal can support you in connecting to and communicating with angels and other celestial entities.

I'd recommend using Celestite when practising breathwork (a therapy that uses the power of the breath to detoxify and nourish the mind, body and soul). Breathing is the most natural action – it's what keeps us alive, after all. Surprisingly enough, most of us aren't breathing properly, which restricts how we function and feel. Using this crystal with breathwork will support you to breathe all the way down towards your stomach and increase your capacity to receive.

*Trust the process*

| | |
|---|---|
| **PHYSICAL HEALING:** | **Believed to relieve fever and lessen inflammation** |
| **CHAKRA:** | **Crown and throat** |
| **SOURCE:** | **USA** |

# CHAROITE

## Courage, surrender, endurance, empowerment

Charoite will help you roll with unexpected twists and turns, so that you can dust yourself off and have the courage to get up and try again. It teaches endurance and perseverance by helping you detach from any negative thoughts that keep you stuck in a rut or repeating old cycles.

If you're drawn to Charoite, it's a sign that you're about to dive deep into your personal development, which will inevitably be a radical ride. It's time to unravel your fears so you can realize your innate superpowers and forgotten talents. Who's really behind the mask that you've been wearing? It's time to take it off so that the world can start getting to know the real you.

This stone will stop your ego getting in the way so you can be more perceptive and objective, instead of taking things personally or projecting your feelings on to a situation. Some huge lessons in compassion and acceptance may be coming your way.

Charoite may help you feel more grounded and focused as you connect more with your spiritual path. It's a stone of psychic self-defence that can reduce distractions and enforce boundaries that stop you feeling drained.

If you're having trouble sleeping, keep a piece of Charoite under your pillow or on your bedside table. It's believed to remedy sleep disorders, including insomnia, sleep paralysis, sleepwalking and nightmares.

*You are stronger than you think. The past needn't have any hold over you*

| | |
|---|---|
| **PHYSICAL HEALING:** | **Said to relieve headaches and migraines and reduce high blood pressure** |
| **CHAKRA:** | **Crown, third eye, solar plexus and base** |
| **SOURCE:** | **Siberia** |

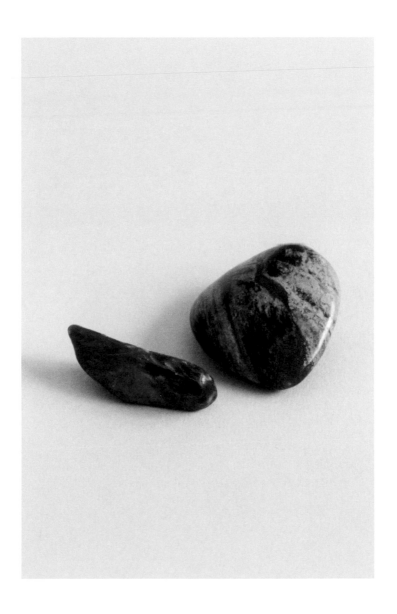

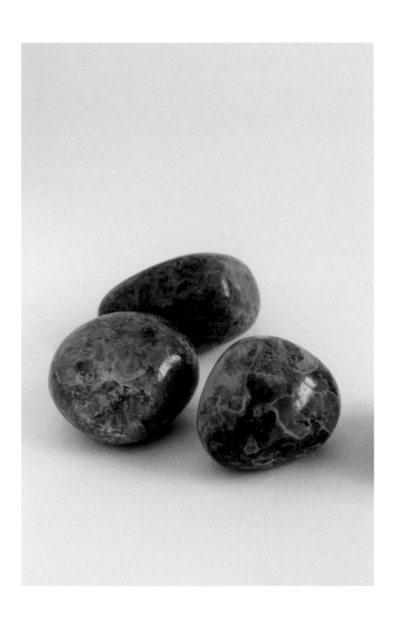

# CHRYSOCOLLA

## Communication, compassion, inspiration, individuality

Sometimes your emotions can come crashing in, like huge waves, and you don't feel you're being heard. These waves are a result of attempts to suppress how you feel until one day they're too strong to ignore. The little things become overwhelming. This could result in having an argument with your lover, being rude to a shop assistant, snappy with a work colleague or impatient with your housemate. Chrysocolla is your permission slip (not that you ever needed one) to be unapologetic in making the call and asking for support. Don't wait until everything gets too much.

This supportive stone will act as an anchor when you're swimming in emotions. Feeling overwhelmed? Chrysocolla can guide you back to reality when you've been in a vortex of compare and despair, misled into thinking you're failing at this wild ride called life when everyone's social media feeds make them look as if they've got it sussed. It's not true. None of us really knows what we're doing: we're all just figuring it out as we go along. It's time to start flowing at your own pace, instead of trying to keep up with what others are doing or following someone else's blueprint.

Chrysocolla is all about helping you find balance and harnessing your emotions so that they can be your guide. Try keeping a journal or doing art therapy to get all of the busy thoughts out of your head so that you can start riding the waves instead of having a total wipe-out. Talk to a therapist or a trusted friend. Let yourself cry. Give your thoughts and feelings space to breathe, release and settle. Hold a piece of Chrysocolla to remember that it's safe to feel it all.

*It's time to dive in and trust yourself and your own feelings*

| | |
|---|---|
| **PHYSICAL HEALING:** | **Believed to balance the thyroid and adrenals, lower high blood pressure and remedy stress, anxiety and panic attacks** |
| **CHAKRA:** | **Throat, heart and base** |
| **SOURCE:** | **Chile, Democratic Republic of Congo, Russia and USA** |

# CITRINE (HEAT-TREATED)

## Confidence, creativity, manifestation, abundance, empowerment

This is the commonest form of Citrine available. It's actually created when Amethyst (page 117) is heated at a high temperature, which changes its colour from purple to yellow-orange, in comparison to natural Citrine's paler, slightly smoky yellow tones. When crystals are formed naturally, they are subjected to high temperatures from within the earth so this process will not damage the crystal, although it will have an effect on its personality.

This type of Citrine is the patron crystal of people-pleasers and procrastinators. Every time you put yourself to the back of the priorities list, life feels a little more lacklustre and those bubbles of anxiety rise to the surface again. Want to rewrite the script? This crystal encourages you to take action for Team You: it's like the cheerleader of the crystal realm.

Cheering you on from the sidelines, Citrine can light the fire in your belly to go for your dreams. It's time to start living by your own rules. Your happiness is the key to success.

*Say yes to your dreams*

| | |
|---|---|
| **PHYSICAL HEALING:** | **Believed to energize, boost metabolism and remedy problems with the back, spine, digestive system, pancreas, liver, spleen and gall bladder** |
| **CHAKRA:** | **Solar plexus** |
| **SOURCE:** | **Man-made in Brazil** |

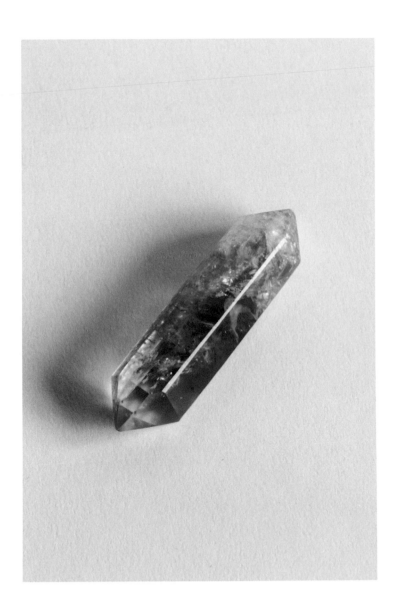

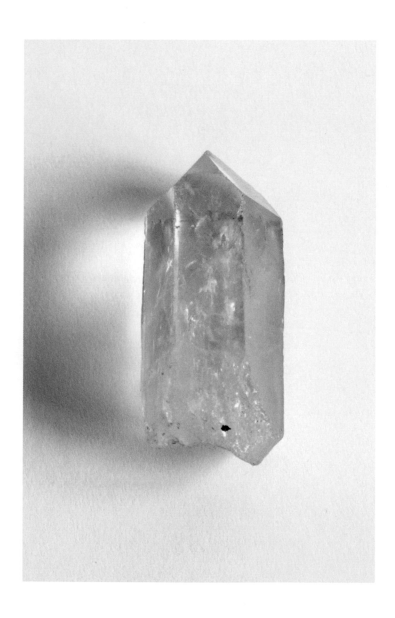

# CITRINE (NATURAL)

## Confidence, new beginnings, abundance, manifestation, optimism

Citrine is an optimistic and energizing crystal. Its name is derived from the French word *citron*, meaning 'lemon', because it's believed to give you a zest for life! It can hoover up negative energy, detoxifying your aura and physical body, and waking you up to fresh opportunities.

This crystal's likely to encourage you to choose the early night instead of a hangover so that you can wake up in the morning ready to seize the day. Citrine's optimistic energy will help you get over a stressful day/week/month or year, so that you can enjoy your downtime without being haunted by work/life responsibilities. If you're focusing on the struggles and hardships of your life, they will distract you from the good things that are happening. There's nothing more demotivating than focusing on the negatives. Although it may not feel like it, wonderful things exist in your life too – you've just forgotten to look for them. Make gratitude your attitude: each day, write down three good things that have happened. This simple exercise (with a little help from Citrine) will make you feel more confident and will guide you to reach your ultimate goal: happiness.

Another tip from Citrine: have a spring clean, tidy your home, declutter your cupboards and put on some fresh bed sheets. Do this to send a signal to the universe that there's space for something new to come into your life.

It's said that Citrine never needs cleansing (see page 27) because it doesn't collect or hold negative energy but a freshen-up is always appreciated.

*Don't be shy – ask for what you want*

| | |
|---|---|
| **PHYSICAL HEALING:** | Believed to energize, boost metabolism and remedy problems with the back, spine, pancreas, liver, spleen, gall bladder and digestive system |
| **CHAKRA:** | Solar plexus |
| **SOURCE:** | France, Madagascar and Russia |

# CLEAR QUARTZ

## Energizing, balancing, manifestation, empowerment

Clear Quartz is one of the commonest and most easily attainable crystals. It's known as the master crystal because of its power to amplify, store, focus, transform and transmit energy. This is why it's synthesized and utilized in so much of our modern technology (see page 20).

If you were stuck on a desert island and could have only one crystal, Clear Quartz would be it. Though it might not get you off the island, it can be programmed (see page 38) to do anything another crystal could. It's like a blank canvas ready to make magic with. All you need to do is ask the Clear Quartz to channel the energy of whatever crystal you choose. You could try it with one of the crystals that has caught your eye in this book and repeat its message three times when you're programming the Clear Quartz crystal.

This high-vibration stone emanates pure white light to help cleanse your energy, balance your chakras and energize your mind, body and spirit. It can bring you into alignment with your highest self.

Clear Quartz is a crystalline battery that can amplify and charge your intentions (see page 78). It can be used for healing, enhancing meditations and dreams, protection, chakra activation, connecting with spirit guides and angels, past-life regression, attracting abundance and pay rises, boosting confidence, all things love related, and so much more.

Use Clear Quartz to activate, harmonize and even supercharge other crystals, like Rose Quartz and Amethyst.

*Clear intention will keep you focused*

| | |
|---|---|
| **PHYSICAL HEALING:** | **Believed to help detoxify, encourage cell regeneration, aid recovery from surgery, balance the energetic system and remedy adrenal fatigue** |
| **CHAKRA:** | **All** |
| **SOURCE:** | **Worldwide, especially Brazil, Madagascar and USA** |

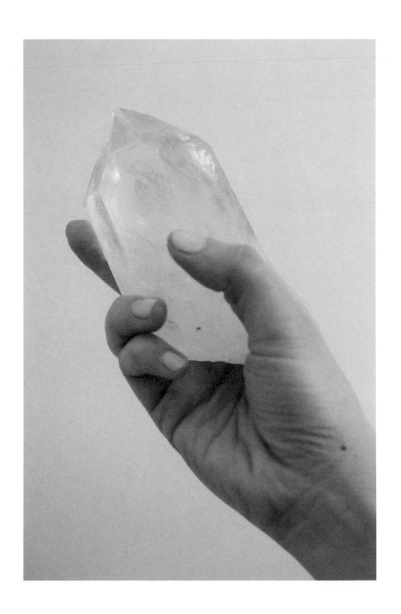

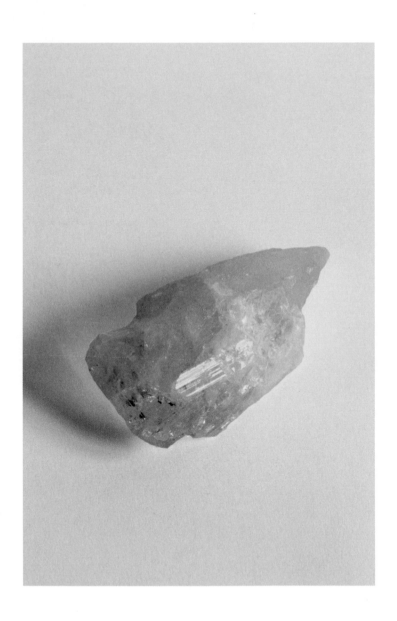

# DANBURITE

## Uplifting, nurturing, expansion, optimism, peace, spiritual evolution

Danburite radiates a soft and tranquil energy that will inspire you to go with the flow. It will make you feel held and supported, soothing your nerves and quieting your mind so that you feel safe to surrender to what's happening in your life.

Working with Danburite enhances spiritual awareness and it has an affinity with Reiki. It can be used as a tool for connecting with your highest self, channelling and connecting with your spirit guides.

This crystal has gentler vibrations than Clear Quartz, while still being potent for purifying and energizing. It's ideal for empaths as it's very calming and supportive.

It's also said to help you to attract like-minded people: if you wear a piece of Danburite when you're dating or at social events, it will help you avoid undesirable attention. You could call it the matchmaker crystal.

Sleeping with a piece of Danburite under your pillow is like a crystalline sedative that can help you drift off with ease.

*Trust that all's good right here, right now*

| | |
|---|---|
| **PHYSICAL HEALING:** | **Thought to resolve blocked energy, which could be the metaphysical root of illness** |
| **CHAKRA:** | **Heart and crown** |
| **SOURCE:** | **Bolivia, Japan, Madagascar, Mexico, Myanmar and Russia. Originally found in Danbury, Connecticut, USA** |

# EMERALD

## Love, compassion, forgiveness, abundance

The earliest known Emerald mines were found in Egypt. Cleopatra, Queen of the Nile, claimed the mines as her own, of course. She had Emeralds crafted into lavish jewellery and possessed a famous collection of crystals. The Ancient Egyptians believed that Emeralds represented rebirth and fertility. In burial ceremonies, a mummy wore an Emerald around their neck as a prayer for eternal youth. It was also used as a protective talisman to ward off evil spirits and spells.

Emerald is a vibrant gemstone that can open the heart to new ways of experiencing love. Finding *the one* isn't always easy and being with *the one* isn't always a smooth ride! Every relationship is a lesson and an opportunity to grow. Emerald may support you to release negative patterns in relationships to create space for more honesty. This is fertile ground to cultivate something more loving and enduring.

Emerald is here to teach you about the power of your own self-worth. Never settle for second best. Harnessing the power of this crystal teaches us that life is abundant and that we're always supported.

When you feel you're ready to check out of Heartbreak Hotel, make an Emerald elixir (page 96) with the intention of opening yourself up to your ultimate vision of love. Write a list of all of the qualities that this person embodies, how you'll feel when you're with them, and the things you imagine doing together – make sure they're all things that you believe to be possible. Get Emerald-clear on how you want to feel in this new relationship so that you can recognize him or her when they find you.

*Relinquish control to receive more love*

| PHYSICAL HEALING: | Believed to heal the heart and improve general well-being |
| --- | --- |
| CHAKRA: | Heart |
| SOURCE: | Africa, Brazil and Russia |

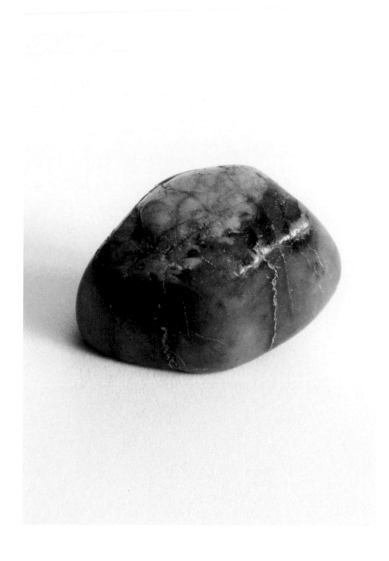

EMERALD

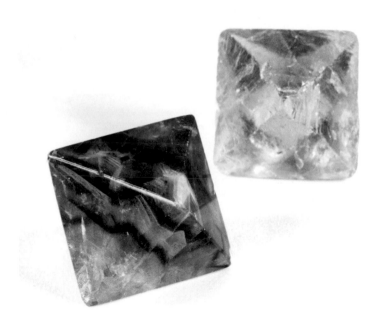

# FLUORITE

## Calming, intuition, protection, wisdom

Fluorite can be found in an array of colours, including purple, green, black, white, yellow, red, pink and clear. A piece may show multiple colours but I've only ever seen it as a purple and green blend. Fluorite is known for its fluorescence: when it's under ultraviolet light it glows.

When your head is in a spin, Fluorite may slow your overactive mind and declutter conflicting thoughts and ideas, bringing order and helping you to avoid a headache or migraine. It can support you in acting on your inspirations and epiphanies with consideration, allowing you to integrate new information strategically instead of acting impulsively. Like a personal assistant, it may stop you rushing ahead and forgetting important details. Keep Fluorite with you to enhance your memory, especially if you're revising or taking exams. It's a useful stone for teachers and students as it supports information retention as well as good communication.

Purple-green Fluorite is one for healers, psychics, tarot readers, mediums, channellers and anyone else who works intuitively. It can create a clear channel for you to access other states of consciousness while simultaneously strengthening your aura so you can be more resilient against unwanted energy. This is definitely one to have in your toolkit for psychic self-defence: it can clear your energy after you've been doing psychic work and remind you to rest so you can avoid burnout.

*Rise above chaos to gain perspective*

| | |
|---|---|
| **PHYSICAL HEALING:** | **Promotes general well-being and self-care; supports the immune system and cellular regeneration** |
| **CHAKRA:** | **Third eye and heart** |
| **SOURCE:** | **Argentina, China, England, Germany and USA** |

# FUCHSITE

## New beginnings, adventure, optimism, collaboration

Fuchsite is a light-hearted and uplifting stone. It will revitalize you and remind you to have fun. It's easy to get caught up in routines and responsibilities but we all need a balance of work *and* play. Are you ready to get this party started? Adventure's calling!

Fuchsite's a stone of new beginnings and optimism. When this stone is around, know that everything will be okay and that the universe has your back. Things are going to get better.

This crystal encourages you to be creative and reminds you that you'll find inspiration when you're embracing all life has to offer. It is a sociable stone that can give you the confidence to go out and meet new people. Say yes to that date. Take a leap of faith and collaborate with others on an inspired endeavour. Get out of your comfort zone.

Super-friendly fuchsite loves to work with other crystals and will amplify the energy of healing grids and layouts (see pages 77 and 90).

*Remember to have fun!*

| | |
|---|---|
| **PHYSICAL HEALING:** | **Believed to support the immune system, reduce inflammation and remedy allergies** |
| **CHAKRA:** | **Heart** |
| **SOURCE:** | **Brazil, India and Russia** |

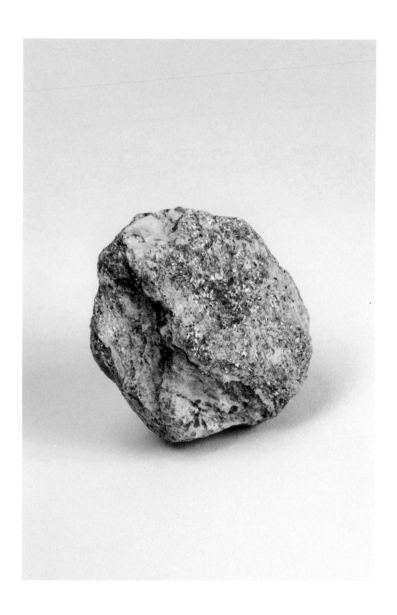

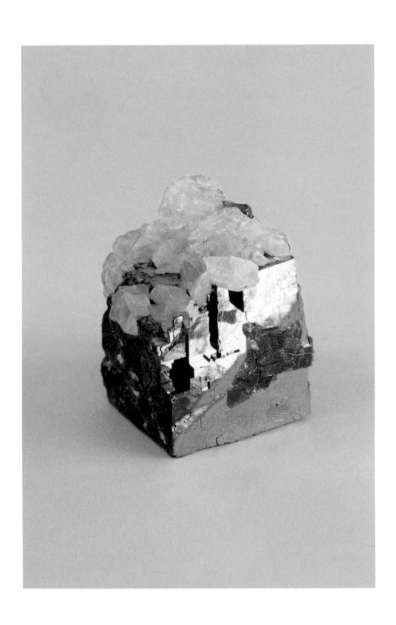

# GALENA*

## Protection, strength, courage, grounding, endurance

Galena will hold your hand as you follow your path through self-development. It can hold space for you to realize life lessons, and dissolve negative frequencies or distractions so that you can create a more fulfilling way of life. This is a time for renewal and new beginnings: make sure that you're patient with yourself so that you can digest the new insights and experiences coming your way. You may feel as if you're being tested as you plunge into the complexity of your emotions. One minute you think you've figured things out, and the next you're flipped upside down, wondering WTF? Work with Galena for strength, courage and endurance. You can do this! It is a stone of independent thinking and will guide you to start leaning into your own answers, instead of following other people's advice.

It's also associated with past-life regression and connecting with ancestral stories, by exploring past lives (this can be done through hypnosis with a therapist, a session with an Akashic Record reader, through a shamanic journey or by listening to a guided meditation). When we uncover patterns and cycles from the past – which may include habits and beliefs that we inherit from our family – we're able to understand what our karma is in this lifetime. This knowledge can help you to realize your life purpose.

Keep Galena close to you if you're spending excessive amounts of time on the computer or around technology. It's believed to absorb electromagnetic pollution, radiation and other forms of damaging environmental energy.

*Be receptive to new experiences and opportunities*

| | |
|---|---|
| **PHYSICAL HEALING:** | **Believed to protect against electromagnetic pollution, as well as the negative effects of chemotherapy and radiation; thought to be a remedy for infections** |
| **CHAKRA:** | **Base** |
| **SOURCE:** | **USA** |

* IMPORTANT: The lead content and other minerals it contains make Galena toxic, so wash your hands after handling. Do not use Galena to make elixirs.

# GARNET (ALMANDINE)*

**Strength, commitment, courage, passion, power, sexuality, vitality**

The word 'garnet' comes from the Latin *granatum*, meaning 'pomegranate', because of its likeness to pomegranate seeds. The pomegranate is a symbol of abundance, fertility/rebirth and marriage in various religions.

Garnet represents empowerment, courage, sensuality and, most of all, commitment. 'Slow and steady wins the race,' says Garnet. It's a grounding and activating stone – you might say it's adaptogenic because it can stabilize and enhance your energy without over-stimulating you.

A stone of lasting love, it's an ally for attracting a new flame or reigniting the spark of a long-term relationship. Wear a Garnet necklace to attract someone who's the full package, lover and best friend, because you want someone who's both. Have this stone crafted into your engagement ring to symbolize passion and commitment.

Garnet is intimately associated with the root chakra, which fuels our primal needs – the sense of survival, security and sexual desire. Working with Garnet will guide you to explore your sexuality and deep intimacy, either within a relationship, solo or somewhere in between.

*Commit to what or who you believe in*

| | |
|---|---|
| **PHYSICAL HEALING:** | **Believed to fortify the immune system and blood, increase metabolism and heal injuries; can be used to support the menstrual cycle and fertility, and to enhance libido and virility** |
| **CHAKRA:** | **Heart and base** |
| **SOURCE:** | **Austria, Brazil, Czech Republic, India and Sri Lanka** |

* IMPORTANT: Do not ingest or use in elixirs.

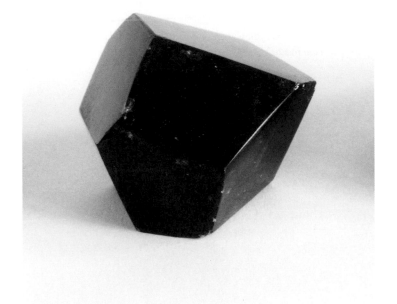

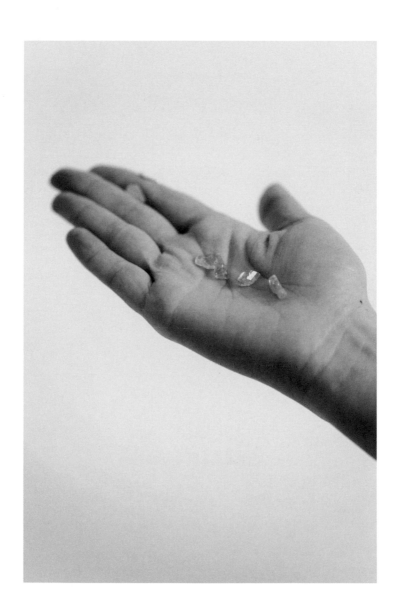

# GOLDEN TOPAZ (IMPERIAL TOPAZ)

## Abundance, law of attraction, manifestation, liberation, creativity

Golden Topaz is a radiant and inspiring crystal. It's like the motivational speaker who wakes you up to a sense of positive entitlement to go for your dreams. Yes, you can do this.

This crystal can tap into your creativity and powers of manifestation. It has the power to reignite the spark of enthusiasm for projects that may have lost their way or been gathering dust because you 'haven't had time'. But when you believe in yourself and take conscious action, the universe will rise up to support you.

Golden Topaz is here to amplify your intention. It's refreshing and liberating, a catalyst for abundance. Keep your eyes on *your* prize. Don't worry about competition or what anyone else is doing.

Allow these golden rays to align you.

*It's your time to step into the spotlight*

| | |
|---|---|
| **PHYSICAL HEALING:** | Believed to balance hormones, support cell regeneration, and remedy urinary and kidney issues |
| **CHAKRA:** | Solar plexus and sacral |
| **SOURCE:** | Africa, Australia, Brazil, Japan, Madagascar, Mexico, Myanmar, Russia, Sri Lanka and USA |

# HAEMATITE

## Protection, grounding, healing, balance, transformation

Haematite is a grounding stone: its energy will flow straight to your root chakra and plug you into the earth. This stone is like a taskmaster, reining in your wandering thoughts when you're struggling to stay focused. Keep a piece of haematite on your desk if you work in a busy environment so that you can stay in the zone. It can help you feel rooted and call back your energy if it's scattered. Working with this stone will help you see your behaviours reflected back to you, and encourage you to take responsibility for your thoughts and actions. It's time to create some new habits and strategies that support you to get the job finished.

If you're going through a transition, like starting a new job or university course, moving house, relocating to a new country or going through a break-up, haematite can filter any anxiety and stress to support you to feel calm and confident as you go through the process. It wants to anchor you in the here and now so you have space to feel what you need to feel. It can help you heal from trauma, grief and abuse, guiding you to rise through crisis stronger and more confident than before.

Airports can have hectic energy: exhaustion from last-minute packing, the moment when you think you've lost your passport (but it's in your back pocket), the hurry to catch a flight, delays, a phobia of flying, nervousness or excitement, then travelling across time zones and eventually acclimatizing to a new environment. This is why jet lag can have such an impact on you. Haematite is the ideal travel companion: keep one in your pocket or tuck a small piece in each sock while you're sitting for the journey, to prevent your energy becoming too unsettled when you're on the move.

*You are strong and supported*

| PHYSICAL HEALING: | Believed to improve blood circulation, blood disorders and heavy menstruation; alleviates pain |
|---|---|
| CHAKRA: | Base |
| SOURCE: | Brazil and USA |

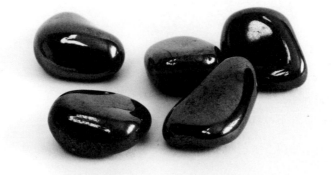

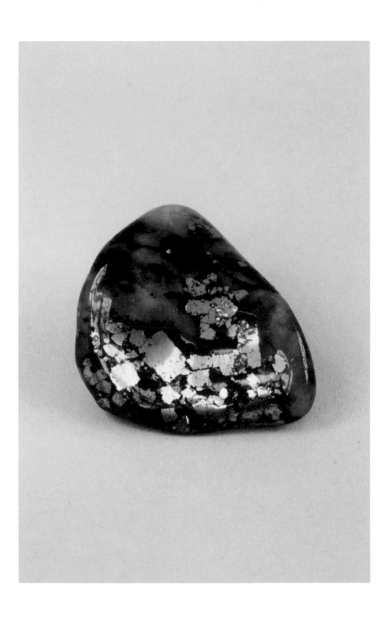

# HEALER'S GOLD

## Confidence, boundaries, grounding, integration, balance, rejuvenation

Healer's Gold is a combination of Pyrite and Magnetite. When you meditate (see page 64) with it or use it in a healing layout (page 90), this stone can help you to absorb new energy and remember any visions or insights you gain from the experience. As its name indicates, it's an ideal stone for healers because it protects the healer's energy during a session and also facilitates the transmission, resulting in both healer and client feeling rejuvenated. Every healer and therapist would benefit from having this crystal in their toolkit. The stone has a strong affinity with Reiki. Healer's Gold will work in synergy with other crystals and facilitate the integration of the crystals' medicine.

Healer's Gold reminds you to set healthy boundaries with your time and energy. Above all, it wants you to appreciate your self-worth and be mindful of how much you do for others. Schedule some time to rest and do things that recharge you, because you can't pour from an empty cup. Allow others to help you, too. Or at least book a massage once a month because you deserve it.

It's an empowering stone that will make you feel more self-assured and guide you to seeing (and receiving) the gold within all of your experiences.

*Nurture yourself and allow time for rest and rejuvenation*

| | |
|---|---|
| **PHYSICAL HEALING:** | **Said to increase general well-being, fortify the blood and give a heightened sense of vitality** |
| **CHAKRA:** | **All** |
| **SOURCE:** | **Arizona, USA** |

# HERKIMER DIAMOND

## Inspiration, creativity, balance, abundance, expansion

Herkimer Diamonds are a type of quartz crystal found in and around Herkimer, New York. They're called Diamonds because that's what they look like. They are usually more affordable.

The double-terminated shape (pointed at both ends) of this crystal means it will simultaneously receive and send energy from different directions. These energies will intersect harmoniously through the body, aligning all of your chakras and supporting energy to flow easily.

Herkimer Diamond can be used for attuning to new frequencies: people, environments and situations. It can support you through transitions when you are integrating new ways of being into everyday life. Wear this crystal if you're starting a new job and getting to know a new team, or you're starting university, moving house or travelling.

This powerhouse can be used to deconstruct scarcity mindsets, when you're worried that there's not enough to go around. This could apply to money, opportunities, time, potential dates, and even worrying that the shoes you've been stalking online will have sold out before payday; you put them on your credit card because you can't live without them, then feel guilty because you can't afford them. Herkimer Diamond can help strengthen your trust muscle to know that we always have what we need and that what we invest in will work out, sometimes in weird and wonderful ways.

Comparison kills creativity: when you're too focused on what you don't have or can't do, you lose sight of other possibilities. Trust that you're always supported, and that's when abundance will channel straight to you.

Herkimer Diamond will magnify the power of other crystals. If you have a small specimen of another stone or you're working with a crystal that has a gentle energy, use Herkimer Diamond to supercharge the other crystal's powers. It's ideal for grids and crystal healing layouts (see pages 77 and 90).

*I am open to inspiration*

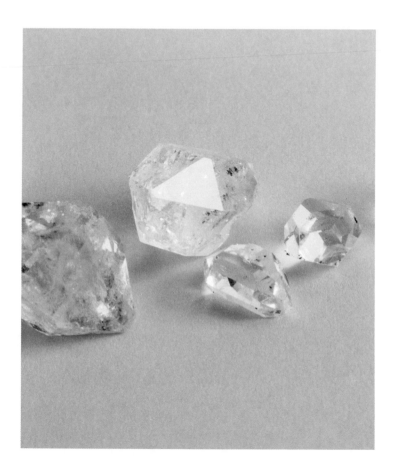

**PHYSICAL HEALING:** Believed to enhance general well-being, protect from radiation, detox the body, enhance energy levels and vitality

**CHAKRA:** Crown and third eye

**SOURCE:** USA

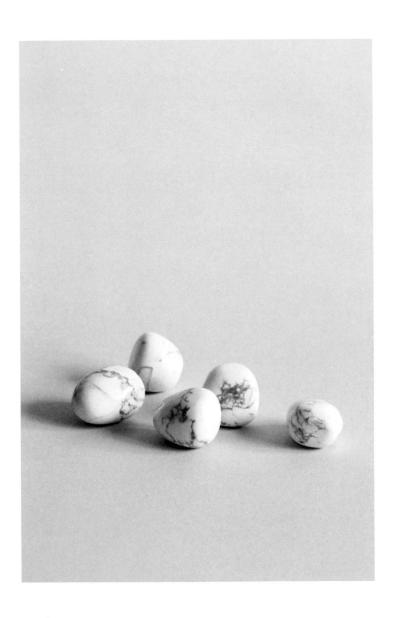

# HOWLITE

## Calming, soothing, overcoming addictions, sleep, protection

Easy, Tiger! Howlite is a protective stone that reduces stress. Its calming energies can slow everything down, stop you overreacting and getting angry or violent.

It's an ally for over-thinkers and those who suffer from anxiety and panic attacks. This stone is ideal to have close by if you work in a busy and demanding environment as it can help you feel centred, despite external distractions and pressures. It can also help you find creative solutions to challenges you thought were impossible.

Howlite's soothing energy can remedy insomnia, supporting you in tuning out of the day's events and never-ending to-do lists.

This stone can also be used to support you in overcoming destructive coping mechanisms, such as alcoholism and smoking, and in seeking the help you need to get through them.

*Time to switch off and take it easy!*

| | |
|---|---|
| **PHYSICAL HEALING:** | **Believed to strengthen bones and teeth, soothe arthritis, rheumatism and toothache, and help the body absorb calcium** |
| **CHAKRA:** | **Crown and solar plexus** |
| **SOURCE:** | **Canada, South Africa and USA** |

# HYPERSTHENE

## Mystical, meditation, protection, subconscious, introspection

Hypersthene is a mystical stone that's known for its visionary powers. Its mesmerizing energy will guide you into a deep, meditative state where you can tune into your subconscious. You'll want it close by when you're meditating or practising yoga. It's like having a shield to protect your energy and ground you, so that you can quieten your mind and be guided into contemplation.

Sometimes the answers are literally hiding in the shadows and may be aspects of yourself you're ashamed of or want to ignore. We all have things we're scared to admit. This doesn't mean you have to speak your fears aloud or make a public declaration. Just being kinder to yourself and learning to accept yourself, despite any perceived 'flaws', can alchemize the shadow – this crystal can help you.

Hypersthene can reveal the truth that was there all along. You just need to be still enough to see it.

*Look within to find the answers*

| | |
|---|---|
| **PHYSICAL HEALING:** | Believed to strengthen the body, fortify the blood and support the internal organs |
| **CHAKRA:** | Third eye, solar plexus and base |
| **SOURCE:** | Australia, Europe, New Zealand and USA |

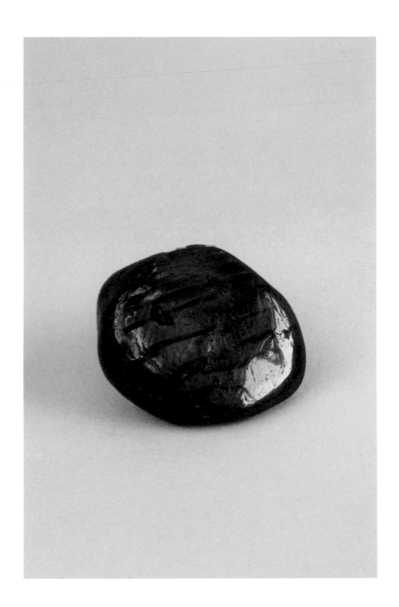

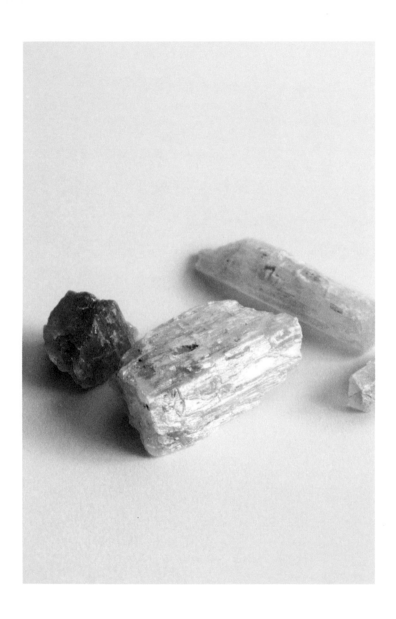

# KUNZITE

## Universal love, kindness, compassion, surrender, forgiveness

Slow down, tender heart. Kunzite's nurturing energy will reassure the vulnerable. For the times when Cupid's playing tricks on you: you've snapped out of the honeymoon haze because your insecurities are bubbling to the surface. This gentle crystal can steer you away from overanalysing every message your lover's sent so that you can tune into the truth. Is this fear or your intuition telling you something's not right? Maybe you feel it's too good to be true so you start sabotaging the relationship because, subconsciously, you feel you don't deserve this kind of love.

When it comes to matters of the heart, Kunzite wants to guide you to heal from heartbreak, betrayal and disappointment. This crystal is like the fairy godmother who will remind you that you deserve to be loved wholeheartedly. So, don't compromise and settle for second best or let the past hold you back.

Meditate (see page 64) with a piece of Kunzite placed on your heart to give this chakra some TLC.

*Choose to see it all with love*

| | |
|---|---|
| **PHYSICAL HEALING:** | **Believed to balance hormones and adrenal glands, support the menstrual cycle and fertility and soothe allergic reactions** |
| **CHAKRA:** | **Heart and crown** |
| **SOURCE:** | **Afghanistan, Brazil, Madagascar and USA** |

# KYANITE – BLUE

## Compassion, forgiveness, justice, truth, communication

Blue Kyanite is a truth-telling crystal. It will guide you to find your voice so that you can use it to share your story. The truth isn't always what you're told: it's what you find out for yourself. This crystal invites you to listen *and* speak up – that's what clear communication is about. We're all entitled to our own version of events, and it's important to have frank discussions, especially with people who hold opposing views, so that we can gain more insight into each other's perspective of the world. When we understand each other and show compassion, we can start bridging gaps to build stronger communities.

Work with Blue Kyanite in matters that require diplomacy and compromise, and to support fair negotiations. Keep it in the office if your team has conflicting ideas: it can open space for everyone to be heard so you can find a creative solution together.

Blue Kyanite is like a peacemaker: it can defuse anger and frustration, bringing calm and clarity, dissolving any confusion or blockages. It will invite you to see the bigger picture so that you can make a positive difference. If you're an activist, public speaker, journalist or researcher, this crystal is for you. It can activate your intuitive superpowers and support you to drop into a meditative state easily. It's like a protective shield to prevent negative influences affecting you.

Like Citrine, Blue Kyanite is said never to need cleansing as such because it doesn't collect or hold negative energy but a freshen-up is always appreciated.

*Listen to your heart and speak your truth*

| | |
|---|---|
| **PHYSICAL HEALING:** | **Believed to support neurological recovery after trauma, stroke or surgery, and to remedy blockages within the body** |
| **CHAKRA:** | **Crown and throat** |
| **SOURCE:** | **Brazil, Kenya, Mexico, Myanmar, South Africa, Switzerland and USA** |

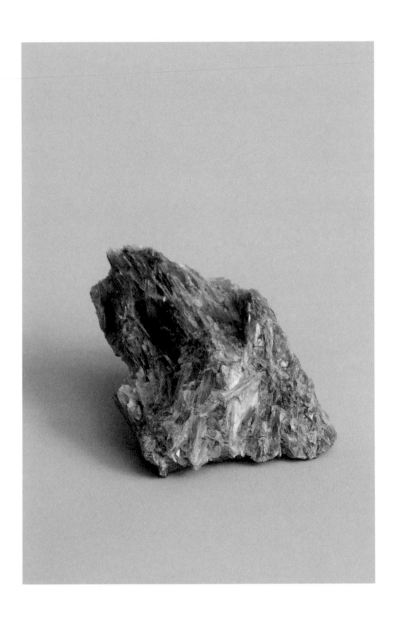

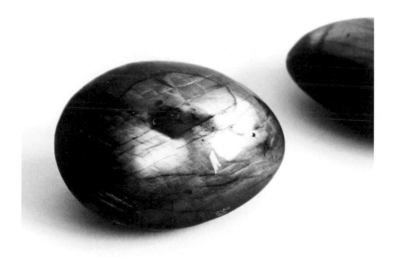

# LABRADORITE

## Protection, grounding, intuition, transformation, creativity

Labradorite is a stone for the mystics, healers, witches, wizards, priestesses, intuitives and creatrixes. It has an affinity with the dark side of the moon and its secrets. It will unveil the hidden truths of the subconscious that are ready to be acknowledged and honoured. This is a stone of self-empowerment, protection, grounding and, ultimately, transformation.

If you're struggling with self-doubt or questioning your life purpose, Labradorite can bring your gaze inwards so that you can dial out from judgement and comparison, then connect with your truth. Take it as your permission to unplug from the usual distractions of modern life so that you can focus on what you want to create and share with the world. Think social-media detox, scheduling dedicated time to working on your craft, setting up an 'out of office' auto-response on your emails, so you don't feel guilty for not replying straight away, and taking time out from socializing. Instead of expecting other people to give you the answers you're looking for, start listening to yourself. Give yourself time and space to explore what's inspiring you.

Labradorite is also associated with the aurora borealis, the Northern Lights, because of the electric flashes you see in it when you move it towards the light.

*Create your own magic!*

| | |
|---|---|
| **PHYSICAL HEALING:** | **Said to remedy chest infections, colds and flu, and to regulate hormones and periods, alleviating PMS** |
| **CHAKRA:** | **All** |
| **SOURCE:** | **Canada, Madagascar, Mexico, Russia and USA** |

# LAPIS LAZULI

## Past lives, intuition, education, communication, problem-solving

Lapis Lazuli is a combination of minerals but for the most part it's Lazurite with Calcite and Pyrite inclusions. Historically, it has been crushed into powder to be used as medicine and to create ultramarine – a pigment that was once prized as highly as gold. Ultramarine was highly sought after by artists because of the iridescent blues it created, giving painting a multidimensional look. Unfortunately, because it was expensive, many couldn't afford to use it or would find themselves in debt before they could finish the painting.

Ancient Egyptians and Babylonians wore Lapis in amulets, pendants and other jewellery because it was known as the 'stone of total awareness', offering protection and insight. I mentioned earlier that Cleopatra wore it as a deep blue eyeshadow glittering with flecks of Pyrite, though it was more than just a beauty statement: it was also believed to enhance spiritual consciousness.

Lapis Lazuli is a visionary stone and will help you develop your intuition, activating your third eye and throat chakras. Enhancing memory and sharpening the mind, it gives you the clarity to find creative solutions to problems.

This majestic stone has an affinity with those who have past-life connections to Ancient Egypt – meditating with it may help you access such memories and support your spiritual evolution during this lifetime. Self-awareness is empowering. It will support you in breaking the chains of self-sabotaging patterns so you can realize your highest potential.

When you align with cosmic consciousness, your intuition is amplified. Be open to receiving guidance from Spirit. You can nourish yourself with wisdom that will offer new opportunities and teach you fresh ways of doing things. Learn about history, science, astrology and esoteric arts. Working with Lapis Lazuli is an invitation to expand your vision of this reality.

*Knowledge is power. Your intuition is your superpower*

| | |
|---|---|
| **PHYSICAL HEALING:** | **Said to alleviate pain and inflammation, soothe headaches and migraines, and support the endocrine and nervous systems** |
| **CHAKRA:** | **Third eye and throat** |
| **SOURCE:** | **Afghanistan, Chile and Russia** |

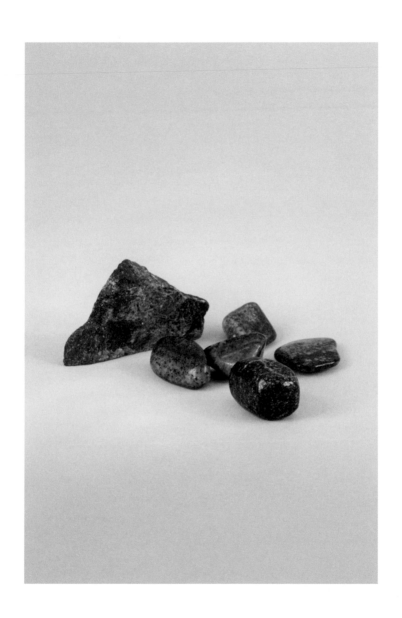

LARIMAR

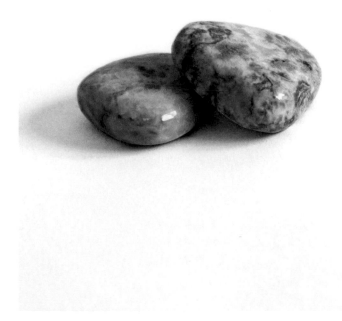

192

# LARIMAR

## Nurturing, emotional healing, intuition, empowerment

If you're looking for a crystal to press pause on your day, choose Larimar. It can calm everything down, defusing any volatile emotions or energies around you. Just like stepping outside and getting some fresh air, it can give you a chance to catch your breath and clear your mind. Once you've had time to recalibrate with Larimar, things can seem different. Lighter. Softer. Quieter. Leaving you feeling mellow.

When you know that you're going to have a potentially stressful day or you're going to be working with an awkward client, keep some Larimar close to you so that you flow with whatever comes up instead of feeling you're fighting a losing battle.

This soothing stone can help you become more fluid with your emotions and tune into your natural rhythms and cycles. Tuning into your feelings is a direct line to accessing your intuition. Feelings aren't facts but they can act as a compass pointing to what you need and what to do. Forget the 'shoulds' and start listening to what your feelings are showing you.

Larimar is associated with the element of water and my piece will always be found in my bathroom because I love using it for ritual baths (see page 104) and literally bathing in its energy.

*Delve within to uncover the true source of your emotions*

| | |
|---|---|
| **PHYSICAL HEALING:** | **Said to be an ally in pregnancy, birth and post-partum; thought to balance hormones and possibly alleviate fever, inflammation and allergic reactions** |
| **CHAKRA:** | **Throat, heart and sacral** |
| **SOURCE:** | **Dominican Republic** |

# LEMURIAN QUARTZ

## Spiritual awakening, intuition, ancient knowledge, meditation

Lemurian Quartz is a unique type of Clear Quartz. The crystals are bright and literally 'crystal clear', with distinguishing ridges on the sides that look like ladders; they represent evolution and past lives. Lemurian Quartz is like the Zen master who reminds us of the steps we need to take to find happiness and spiritual enlightenment.

Lemurian Quartz is associated with legends of an ancient civilization called Lemuria, a lost land in the South Pacific that's believed to have existed fourteen thousand years ago. Lemuria was said to have been a highly intuitive and heart-centred society. As the story goes, the Lemurians predicted that a great flood was coming so the priests and prophets stored information in crystals to safeguard the knowledge of their culture. When the flood came, the crystals were sown like seeds into the earth so they'd be found and used to access the wisdom of the Lemurians for healing, clairvoyance and following the path of enlightenment. These crystals are believed to carry the memories of this lost world, knowledge that was intended for use in support of the greater good in these modern times.

Lemurian Quartz crystals have a high-frequency vibration and own the potential to support accelerated personal development, expanding your consciousness to remind you of your interconnectedness. They're powerful and can be used as a gateway to connect with Lemurian wisdom as well as spirit guides, celestial realms and your highest self. Lemurian Quartz is definitely one to supercharge your meditations as it will activate all of your chakras so that you're a clear channel for spiritual downloads, in the form of inspiration, visions, messages and insights.

Lemurian Quartz crystals can teach you how powerful your intentions are and prove that beliefs create your reality. Getting to know this crystal will open you up to new ways of experiencing life.

*What wisdom can you find from connecting to other realms?*

| | |
|---|---|
| **PHYSICAL HEALING:** | **Supports well-being and mental clarity, radiation therapies and chemotherapy; brings strength to the physical body** |
| **CHAKRA:** | **Crown, third eye and heart** |
| **SOURCE:** | **Brazil** |

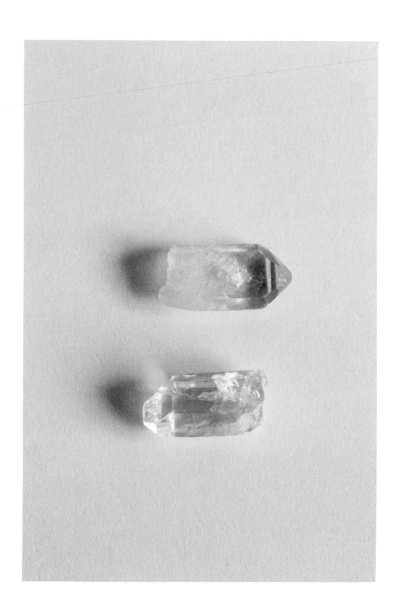

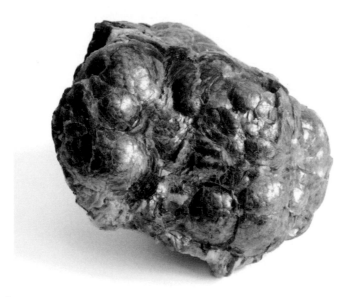

**PHYSICAL HEALING:** Said to support brain function and help you feel uplifted, as it has the subtle energies of lithium

**CHAKRA:** Third eye, heart and throat

**SOURCE:** Africa, Brazil, Greenland and USA

# LEPIDOLITE*

## Nurturing, calming, overcoming addictions and anxiety, sleep

Take a seat and let's talk it out. Lepidolite is like the therapist of the crystal realm. When you're with this stone it's as if you're sitting on a therapist's sofa and they're asking you all of the right questions to decipher what's going on in your head. It's got the perfect bedside manner that can make you feel safe and supported. This stone's soothing energy will invite you to slow down and be present in the moment so you can be more accepting of what's really going on. Especially when your mind is distorting your view of reality. Lepidolite has a tendency to remind us that the more you over-think life, the more elusive the answers become. If you're caught up on the how, what, when and why, or forcing yourself to move forward and overanalysing every option, it just makes things complicated when the answer is so simple: stop and take it all one step at a time. Wondering what your life purpose is? It's to live each day wholeheartedly, doing what you love.

If you're unsure of an opportunity that's come your way, like a new job, collaboration or the chance to relocate to another city, Lepidolite can help you to zone into your gut instinct or intuition. Think of scenario A and scenario B – to do or not to do: instead of weighing up the logical pros and cons, close your eyes and feel how your body reacts when you imagine yourself in the different scenarios. In scenario A, perhaps you can feel butterflies fluttering inside you; scenario B may feel tight and restrictive. Which would you choose? Tune into your body's natural responses: they're signposts to the answers you're looking for.

You can never make the wrong decisions: every choice you make guides you towards getting to know yourself better and this crystal can assist you.

Lepidolite has a high lithium content. Lithium-based medicines are widely used to treat psychological conditions. Do not consume it in any form unless it's prescribed for you by a doctor.

Spend some time with Lepidolite, meditate with it, sleep with it under your pillow. When you slow down, the epiphanies will start rolling in. Keep it by your bed if you're experiencing sleep disorders, such as insomnia, caused by stress and anxiety, or nightmares and sleep paralysis.

*Live in the present moment – it's OK not to have all the answers right away*

* IMPORTANT: Do *not* ingest or use in elixirs.

# MALACHITE*

## Protection, transformation, love, emotional empowerment

Malachite is like a battery that recharges your heart so that you feel safe to love again. It is all about plugging you into feelings of unconditional love, reminding you that, yes, you are 100 per cent lovable. We're all perfectly imperfect and this stone gives us the courage to be ourselves, without having to censor who we are to be attractive to another person or to fit in with a group. Keep Malachite with you when you're going on a date or meeting new people, like your potential in-laws. Working with this stone may guide you to become more aware of your emotional triggers so that self-awareness can guide you through challenging situations or growth opportunities. If you find yourself arguing with your partner, family or friends, Malachite can nudge you to see your role in the conflict. Relationships aren't always as they're depicted in the movies: they can be messy and bring up all sorts of insecurities.

Malachite can always encourage you to take responsibility for your actions and be compassionate. Let your ego take a back seat and put your heart behind the driving wheel.

As a tumbled stone, Malachite has unique patterns that look like atolls – just check out aerial pictures of the Maldives to see what I mean. These formations also look like eyes, which is why Malachite is thought of as a tool for enhancing visionary powers and as a guard against negative intentions. It's said this stone will warn you of danger by breaking into pieces.

Malachite is believed to protect against radiation by absorbing negative energy. This is why it needs regular cleansing to allow its energy to flow efficiently. Do not use the salt-water cleansing method, though, as it will damage the finish of this crystal.

*You can awaken your visionary powers and intuition*

| | |
|---|---|
| PHYSICAL HEALING: | Thought to support the immune system and recovery from illness and surgery; believed to reduce inflammation, alleviate pain and enhance well-being and vitality |
| CHAKRA: | Heart, throat, solar plexus |
| SOURCE: | Australia, Chile, Democratic Republic of Congo, South Africa and USA |

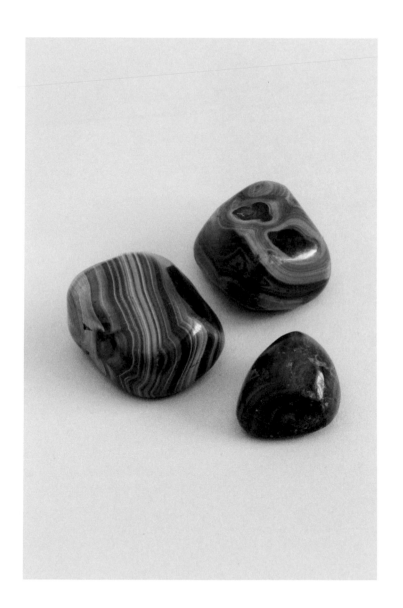

* IMPORTANT: Do *not* ingest or use in elixirs.

MOLDAVITE

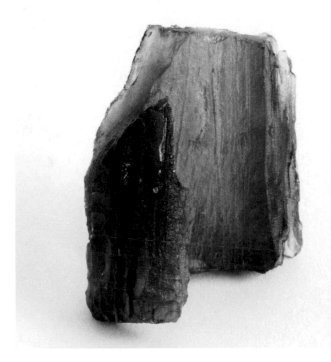

**PHYSICAL
HEALING:**   Said to guide you towards understanding the root
cause of imbalances or physical disease

**CHAKRA:**   Third eye and heart

**SOURCE:**   Czech Republic

# MOLDAVITE

## Transformation, spiritual awareness, grounding, healing

Moldavite is a tektite that formed when a meteor collided with the earth more than 14 million years ago and can only be found in the Czech Republic. It's associated with the legends of the Holy Grail and is highly prized for its metaphysical gifts. It's a hybrid talisman for transformation because it is a fusion of earth and extraterrestrial origin.

Lots of people report this stone to be a game changer and catalyst in their spiritual awakening. You could think of it as the ayahuasca of the crystal realm. Ayahuasca is a plant medicine that's native to the Amazon: it's taken ceremonially and can induce energetic emotional and physical purging. Moldavite will propel you to upgrade your life in ways you'd never imagine, including heightening your sense of connectivity and compassion to the world around you, having the confidence to make some radical changes to your lifestyle and being hyperaware of synchronicities popping up in your day.

Because of its intensity, you're advised to take a few days to acclimatize to this stone's energy before prolonged use. You could begin with short doses of meditation (ten to twenty minutes) with it before you start wearing it or keeping it with you during the day.

When you're lost in thoughts too much, bring Moldavite's medicine to your life by going outside and connecting with nature. Hug a tree. Forest bathe. Feel your bare feet on the grass, rooted into the ground, and reach your arms up to the sky to draw nature's energy into your body from both sky and earth. Become really rooted and notice how your anxiety and stress dissipate. Do this with Moldavite in one hand to amplify the experience.

If you can't get outdoors, you can try this visualization exercise instead: lie down somewhere comfortable and place Moldavite on your heart chakra or third eye, then imagine being rooted to the earth and reaching your hands up to the heavens.

Moldavite fills you with a deep sense of love and reminds you of the importance of looking after the planet, preserving its ecosystem so we can continue enjoying its abundance.

*You are an intrinsic and important part of the universe; you can make a difference*

# MOONSTONE

## Cycles, change, new beginnings, inspiration, creativity, intuition

Moonstone is associated with the moon and feminine energies. It will guide you to tune into your natural cycles and rhythms, as well as turning up the volume to your intuition.

For those times when your creative flow feels as dry as the Sahara desert, inspiration has become as fleeting as a mirage, and there's no room on your to-do list to bring anything to life – not as you want to, anyway – get yourself some Moonstone ASAP.

Ignoring your vital need to rest and recharge will send you on an orbit to burnout, leaving no juice for any kind of creativity. Moonstone encourages you to feel and acknowledge what you need to feel supported so that you can keep the muse on your side. There are some great apps available to track your menstrual cycle, which allow you to start recording your energy levels; when you do this regularly you'll see patterns emerging. You'll get to know the days when you're likely to feel like Wonder Woman or Superman and others when you just want to nap and watch Netflix. These pearls of wisdom will help you manage your life so that you can schedule according to your energy levels, and no longer feel as if you're trying to swim against the current.

Know when you need to step out of the hustle. All those feelings you're experiencing are trying to communicate something to you. When you create space for yourself to press pause on life, you open yourself up to epiphanies and breakthroughs.

It's time to start flowing with the blessings the universe is showering you with, instead of feeling sidetracked.

*Your feelings are your guide. Honouring your cycles will set you free*

| | |
|---|---|
| **PHYSICAL HEALING:** | **Believed to assist fertility and menstrual cycles, plus the thyroid, pituitary, breasts and hormones in general; used for recovery after operations on breasts and womb** |
| **CHAKRA:** | Crown, third eye and sacral |
| **SOURCE:** | India, Myanmar, Sri Lanka and USA |

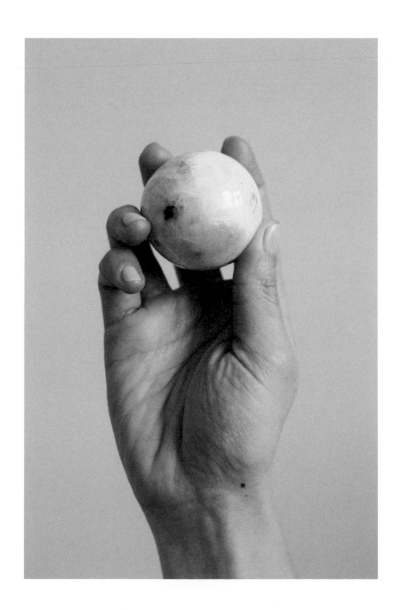

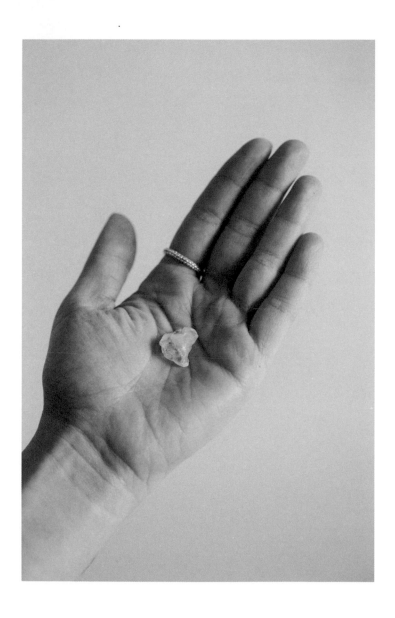

# MORGANITE

## Divine love, surrender, compassion, liberation

Morganite has a delicate and uplifting energy that radiates divine love. Tuning into the frequencies of this crystal can align you to higher dimensions of love and light. If you were to visualize a peony as it blooms, each petal unfurling until it looks like a voluptuous love bomb, Morganite can have the same effect on your heart chakra. Its serene and nurturing presence reminds us to stay soft, especially after a trauma, abuse, heartbreak or grief, to allow the process to flow as it needs to. It wants you to be kind to yourself and take as much time and space as you need.

The energy of this crystal reminds me of the feeling after you've been on the best holiday ever with your partner, family or friends, to a retreat or a festival. Like you're all kindred spirits and you've just had the most incredible time making memories. You almost don't want it to end. It's all about remembering the good times (and the promise of more). Morganite is a dose of exactly that.

It wants to teach you what it is to truly love and be loved, without attachments or conditions. When you choose to surrender the attachment to toxic and unresolved relationships, you give yourself permission to heal and move forward.

Meditating with Morganite may attune you to higher states of consciousness and assist you in connecting with angels, spirit guides and ascended beings for extra support and guidance.

*Keep your heart soft and open to love*

| | |
|---|---|
| **PHYSICAL HEALING:** | **Said to support the nervous system and remedy heart disorders** |
| **CHAKRA:** | **Heart** |
| **SOURCE:** | **Africa, Brazil, Madagascar and USA** |

# OBSIDIAN – BLACK

## Protection, cleansing, grounding

Black Obsidian is volcanic glass and is a powerful stone for protection. It acts as a shield to negativity and can be used for psychic self-defence, especially when you sense someone projecting unwanted vibes your way. This could be someone who's trolling you online, a bully at the office, a jealous friend or an 'it's complicated' ex. Black Obsidian will help you cut ties that have been draining your energy so that you can start focusing on moving forward.

Are you ready to let go of what's been holding you back? If Black Obsidian has found its way to you then the answer is most definitely yes. It can act as your bodyguard, and support you in setting yourself free from negative attachments, unresolved relationships and destructive habits. This might be deleting the number of an ex you keep hooking up with, getting help from a therapist to overcome an addiction or looking for a job that showcases your talents. It's time to get real and start walking your talk.

Working with Black Obsidian will help you understand the lessons your experience has taught you so you can move forward, feeling more empowered and stronger than before.

Call back your power.

Surrender regrets and disappointment.

Forgive the past to move forward.

You're wiser now.

*It's time to see the truth of your situation and be empowered by the past*

| | |
|---|---|
| **PHYSICAL HEALING:** | **Believed to alleviate pain and support recovery from shock, trauma and abuse** |
| **CHAKRA:** | **Base** |
| **SOURCE:** | **Argentina, Armenia, Australia, Azerbaijan, Canada, Chile, El Salvador, Georgia, Greece, Guatemala, Iceland, Italy, Japan, Kenya, Mexico, New Zealand, Papua New Guinea, Peru, Scotland, Turkey and USA** |

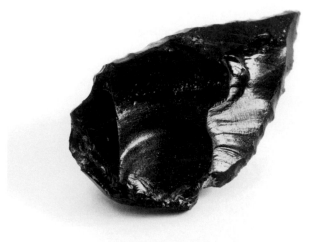

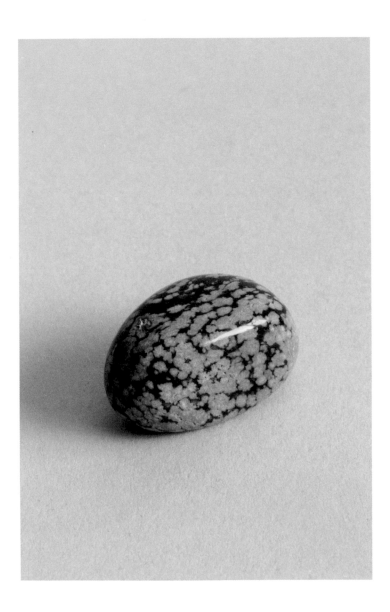

# OBSIDIAN - SNOWFLAKE

## Change, boundaries, balance, grounding

Snowflake Obsidian is an insightful crystal that can guide you to be more decisive and confident in your purpose. What's holding you back from living life on your terms? Are you always making compromises for other people's needs/demands? How long have you been waiting for X, Y or Z to happen so you can take that bold leap of faith?

This crystal will ground and support you, balancing your mind, body and spirit so you can tune into the best choice for *you*, instead of reacting to stress, anxiety, peer pressure, guilt or FOMO (fear of missing out). It has the power to protect you from those who are trying to manipulate you.

This pretty stone is here to guide you to be more objective and less emotionally charged, leading you towards what will nurture your needs and goals

Listen to your intuition instead of the 'shoulds'. What are you ready to let go to make space for the new? Take some time to process your realizations. Talk things over with someone you trust. Visualize your desired outcome; use your imagination to try it on for size before you make any moves. Meditate or spend time recording your thoughts to gain perspective.

Be open to new possibilities.

You've waited long enough to make some (overdue) changes.

It's time to start living by your own rules so that you can feel fulfilled.

*It's OK to trust your intuition and put yourself first*

| | |
|---|---|
| **PHYSICAL HEALING:** | **Believed to alleviate pain, support recovery from shock, trauma and abuse; said by some to prevent cancer cells dispersing through the body, although this has not been scientifically proven** |
| **CHAKRA:** | **Third eye and base** |
| **SOURCE:** | **Mexico** |

# OPAL

## Inspiration, emotional intelligence, intuition

Opal is famous for its flashes of 'fire' and iridescent colours. This eye-catching stone will make you feel as if you're living in technicolour. It's said to bring inspiration and adventure to whoever owns it. It can awaken your innate psychic abilities, opening your third eye to decipher what your intuition is guiding you towards.

Associated with the elements of water and fire, Opal may stir up your emotions and passions. It can heighten your sense of perception, and attuning to this crystal will help you identify perpetuating cycles that need to be cleared and resolved so you can break the cycle and start fresh.

There are rumours that Opal is unlucky. The idea came from *Anne of Geierstein*, a novel by Sir Walter Scott! It's not based on an experience or ancient belief. The lead character, Lady Hermione, was accused of being a demoness. She wore an enchanted Opal in her hair. When she was angry the Opal would flash fiery red, and when she was happy it would sparkle. On one fateful day, drops of holy water fell on the stone and Lady Hermione became ill. The next day all that was found of her and the Opal was a pile of dust. Hence Opal's bad reputation, which devastated trade for almost fifty years.

From my own experience, Opal's energy can feel like a whirlwind, sometimes leaving me feeling overwhelmed. If you notice yourself feeling unsettled after spending time with this stone, I'd recommend having a break from it and working with a grounding crystal like Black Tourmaline or Haematite.

*My feelings are guiding me towards something wonderful*

| | |
|---|---|
| **PHYSICAL HEALING:** | **Believed to improve brain function and eyesight, balance hormones after childbirth and support new mothers in breastfeeding their babies*** |
| **CHAKRA:** | **All** |
| **SOURCE:** | **Australia, Brazil, Guatemala, Honduras, Japan, Peru and USA** |

* Do not give small stones to babies.

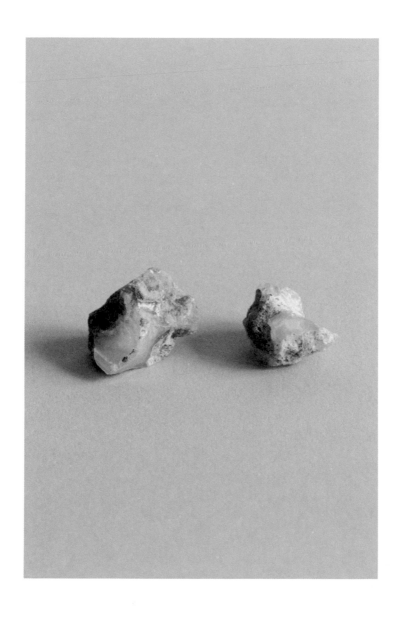

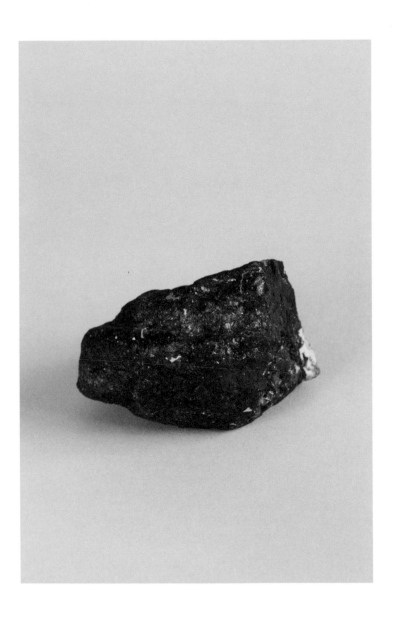

# PEACOCK ORE
# (CHALCOPYRITE, BORNITE)

## Confidence, renewal, abundance, self-expression, empowerment

Most of us have a sparkly, shimmery, bright and extravagant item of clothing tucked somewhere in the wardrobe. It's usually reserved for festivals and fancy-dress parties or getting moth-eaten waiting for a 'special' occasion. Whenever you wear it, you feel incredible, and it's like your superhero uniform. Y'know that feeling? Well, it pretty much sums up how Peacock Ore will make you feel, except you can wear it at any time and know you won't get strange glances on the bus. This stone wants you to show off your true colours, regardless of the occasion. Keep a piece in your handbag for a night out, a date or an interview to boost your confidence.

Let your hair down! Peacock Ore is a nudge to be spontaneous and have fun. It wants you to dance like no one's watching. Sometimes it's better to go with the flow instead of making plans.

For wardrobe-malfunction days, when you can't choose an outfit that feels right (we all have them), accessorize with some Peacock Ore so that you feel confident in whatever you're wearing – even if none of it matches.

Peacock Ore inspires joy and creativity, giving you the impetus to take action towards your dreams. When you feel confident and empowered, you're magnetic. You become a direct line to new opportunities and synchronistic happenings. You're so ready for this!

*Life is fun and you're invited to enjoy the ride!*

| PHYSICAL HEALING: | Believed to improve adrenal function, balance metabolism, reduce fevers and prevent contagious illnesses |
|---|---|
| CHAKRA: | All |
| SOURCE: | Kazakhstan and Mexico |

# PYRITE (FOOL'S GOLD)*

## Prosperity, manifesting, logic, power, action, focus, confidence

Pyrite is a protective and grounding stone. It has a masculine energy that reminds me of the Emperor in the tarot. It's all about getting down to business, checking the details and taking action. You need to anchor all of your ideas with a strategy so that they can come to life.

Forget Red Bull giving you wings: meditating with Pyrite can give you an instant energy boost and do wonders for your self-esteem. This stone incites confidence, commitment and going for gold! There's nothing foolish about Pyrite.

This shiny stone may increase your perception of motives, stimulate your intellect and freshen up your memory.

It's an ideal stone for business and manifesting your goals as it encourages you to be assertive with your intentions and take considered action.

Holding Pyrite at the end of a meditation will assimilate high-vibrational energies into your body and plug you back into the here and now.

*Action speaks louder than words*

| | |
|---|---|
| **PHYSICAL HEALING:** | **Said to fortify the immune system, alleviate blood disorders and remedy male impotence and infertility** |
| **CHAKRA:** | **Solar plexus** |
| **SOURCE:** | **France, Italy, Japan, Norway, Peru, Russia and Spain** |

* IMPORTANT: Pyrite is *not* safe to ingest or use in elixirs.

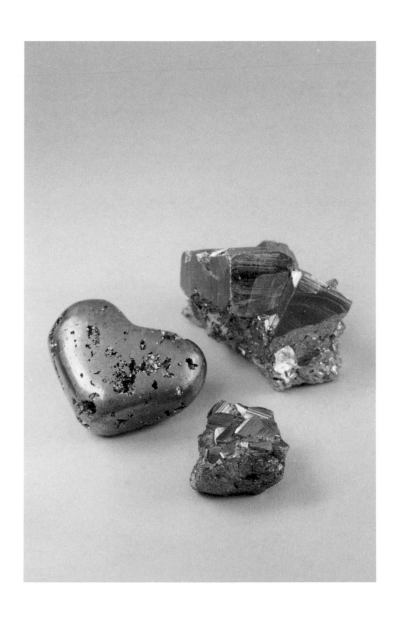

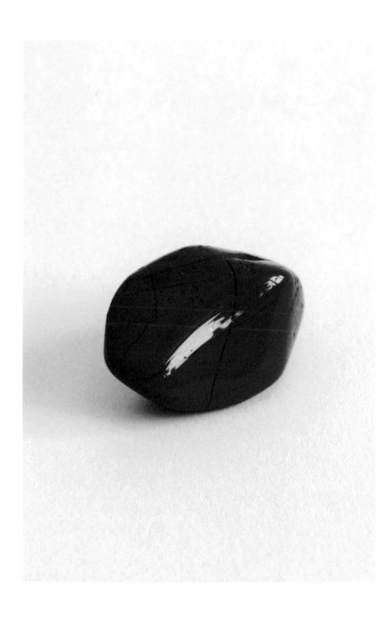

RED JASPER

# RED JASPER

## Confidence, empowerment, stamina, boundaries, energy

Red Jasper's powers are steady and gradual. It can help you to take things in your stride and feel grounded through life's changes and challenges. It's a stimulating crystal that imbues you with confidence and a sense of purpose.

When working with Red Jasper, you will be encouraged to set balanced boundaries around your time, space and energy. Think of streamlining your ever-evolving to-do list. Doing a lot but don't feel like you're getting anywhere? It's time to get organized and objective. Prioritize. Have a life audit and say no to the things that are holding you back.

Know what works for you. Schedule in more time to do what you love and delegate things that are less important. This is when you'll begin to see tangible results for all of your efforts.

Red Jasper is an empowering stone that can support single parents who need to play mother and father roles. Like all red stones, it embodies commitment and passion and can make you feel more sensual and sexual.

*Take your time to build foundations*

| | |
|---|---|
| **PHYSICAL HEALING:** | Thought to increase physical strength and stamina, fortify the blood and immune system, assist recovery from heart surgeries, increase fertility and support IVF treatment |
| **CHAKRA:** | Solar plexus and base |
| **SOURCE:** | Brazil, France, Germany, India, Russia and USA |

# RHODOCROSITE

## Support, connection, love, surrender

Rhodocrosite is like the big sister/brother/best friend of the crystal realm. It has the power to open your heart and make you feel supported through times when you're feeling overwhelmed by everyday life, stress, heartbreak, trauma or abuse.

Reach out and ask for help. You don't have to go through this alone. When you hold tight on your feelings, you limit how much love you're able to receive. Sometimes all you need is for someone to listen to your worries. As soon as you say them aloud, those worries will lose their power as if by magic. But this isn't magic: it's all about connection. Connection will lighten the burden and help you to see things differently, with a fresh perspective. This stone will guide you to see a way out so you don't have to feel stuck any more.

Your problems may not be solved overnight but they have a better chance of being relieved when you talk to someone trustworthy about how you're feeling.

You are loved. You are supported. You are courageous.

You'll get through this.

*Allow yourself to be supported*

| | |
|---|---|
| **PHYSICAL HEALING:** | **Said to support the heart, improve blood circulation, lower blood pressure and alleviate stress-related conditions** |
| **CHAKRA:** | **Heart** |
| **SOURCE:** | **Argentina, China, Japan, Peru, South Africa and USA** |

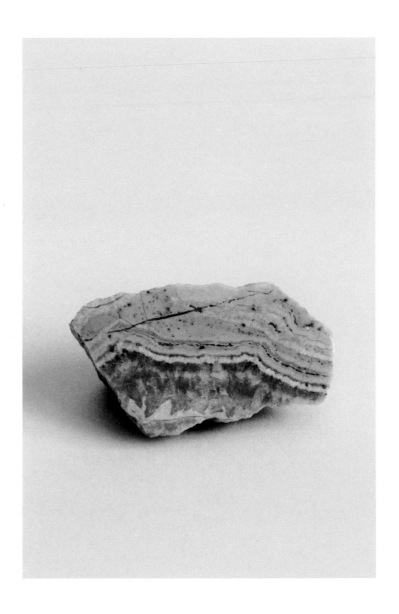

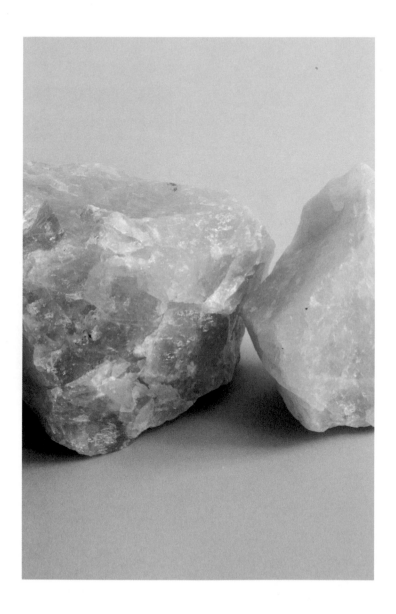

# ROSE QUARTZ

## Love, compassion, forgiveness, calm, support, surrender

Rose Quartz is the famous 'love stone'. It may be an obvious choice if you're looking for *the one* but just taking a piece of this crystal everywhere you go won't attract a lover. Ultimately, Rose Quartz wants to align you to self-appreciation and self-love, because true love starts with you. There's a saying by Rumi that sums this up beautifully: 'Your task is not to seek for love, but merely to seek and find all the barriers within yourself that you have built against it'.

How much love are you allowing yourself to receive in *every* aspect of your life? Rose Quartz can bring harmony to your existing relationships – friendships, family, professional and romantic – and, if you're single, potentially guide you to meet someone who's really aligned with your highest intentions, if that's what you want to call in.

But the relationship with yourself is the most vital of them all. As you learn to love yourself, you'll have so much more to give. Change begins with love.

Rose Quartz is like a huge hug. It'll ground you and slow everything down, helping you mellow out and be kind and compassionate to yourself. This pink stone helps you stay in the present moment, your worries fading away. It'll also teach forgiveness – for others and *yourself* – and open your heart to receiving more love.

*The love you've been seeking has always been inside. When you find it in yourself, you find it in others*

| | |
|---|---|
| **PHYSICAL HEALING:** | **Believed to soothe skin, headaches and other stress-related conditions, support fertility and heal post-partum mothers after complicated births** |
| **CHAKRA:** | **Heart** |
| **SOURCE:** | **Brazil, Madagascar, Namibia, South Africa and USA** |

# RUBY

## Confidence, power, love, sensuality, commitment

The Ruby has been treasured throughout history as a status symbol for power, passion and prosperity. It can encourage you to be more headstrong and determined: it's time to start believing in yourself. This crystal will help turn down doubt so that you can be more confident in your decisions. Say 'yes' to inspiring opportunities that come your way. Step into your power. Your mission is to dare greatly to become the ultimate version of yourself. Wear Ruby to connect with your higher purpose and for energetic attraction. This crystal can fill you with a sense of unstoppable life-force energy; remember to take days off in your quest for world domination to avoid burnout.

To all lovers, Ruby is also a famous talisman for love, sensuality and loyalty. It may amplify your powers of seduction and inspire deep intimacy. Ancient Egyptian dancers would wear Ruby in their navel to enhance their sex appeal. Wear this crystal if you want to explore new territory with your lover or reignite a spark that's been fading.

*You are (more than) enough (always)*

| | |
|---|---|
| **PHYSICAL HEALING:** | **Thought to improve circulation, immunity and support heart disorders, as well as improve fertility, virility and libido** |
| **CHAKRA:** | **Base** |
| **SOURCE:** | **Brazil, India, Myanmar, Sri Lanka, Thailand and USA** |

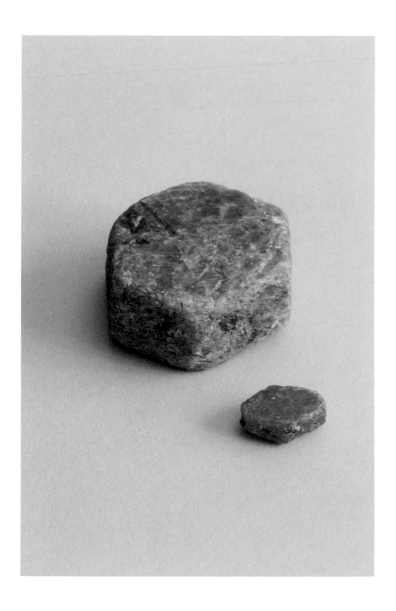

223

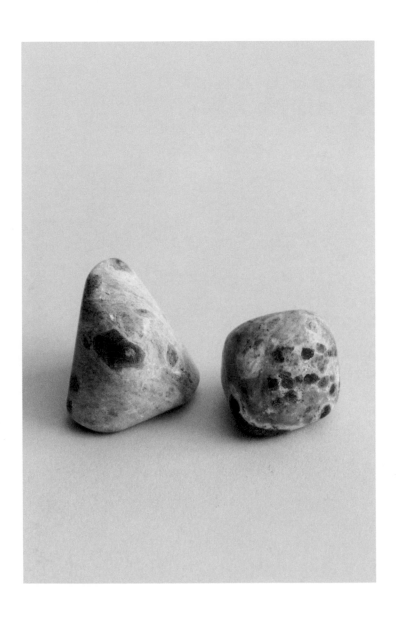

# RUBY IN FUCHSITE

## Courage, self-love, strength

In this fusion stone, the passionate and courageous energies of Ruby are blended with the soothing and nurturing energies of Fuchsite, making this a dynamic, heart-centred crystal. Its potent medicine can rejuvenate mind, body and spirit.

It calls you to check-in with yourself and become more self-reliant, to listen to your needs and desires. This is where you'll find fulfilment. Let go of fear and expectations. Be bold and put yourself out there. Wake up the love warrior within you by bringing your awareness into the here and now. Ruby in Fuchsite will support you to grow through vulnerability, leading to more intimacy and empowerment.

Step into love wholeheartedly. See also Ruby (page 222) and Fuchsite (page 166).

*Shine bright and follow your heart*

| | |
|---|---|
| **PHYSICAL HEALING:** | **Believed to enhance a general sense of well-being and support recovery after illness** |
| **CHAKRA:** | **Heart and base** |
| **SOURCE:** | **India** |

# RUTILATED QUARTZ

## Abundance, manifestation, focus, activating

Rutilated Quartz is Clear or Smoky Quartz with the inclusion of Rutile, which gives it the appearance of metallic threads darting through the crystal. Some say it's angel's hair, while others believe it's the hair of the Roman goddess of love, Venus. Either way, this is a crystal that encapsulates something divine that may help you learn some spiritual truths along the way.

Like all quartzes, Rutilated Quartz will amplify your thoughts and stimulate your energetic system by healing emotional blocks and releasing stagnant energy. The Rutile within this stone brings order and will help you focus your intentions. It's a wonderful crystal to have on your desk if you're easily distracted and your thoughts wander from anything to do with work. If you're a social-media addict and you've become a scrolling zombie, get some Rutilated Quartz to help you focus on the things that you actually need to be doing.

Work with this crystal to accelerate the process of manifestation, healing, spiritual awakening and psychic development.

*Energy flows where intention goes*

| | |
|---|---|
| **PHYSICAL HEALING:** | **Believed to help respiratory infections and disorders, and possibly to stimulate hair growth and prevent loss** |
| **CHAKRA:** | **All** |
| **SOURCE:** | **Brazil and Madagascar** |

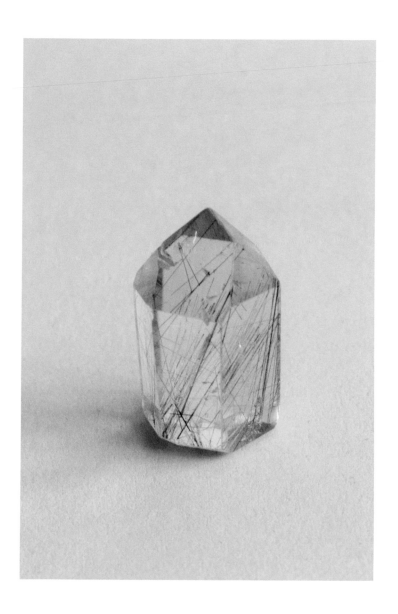

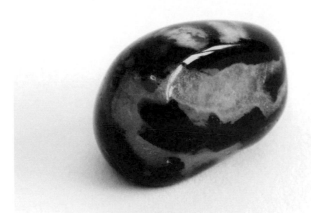

# SARDONYX

## Confidence, leadership, courage, uplevelling, boundaries

Sardonyx is an empowering stone that will encourage you to be more confident. It will guide you to find the inner strength needed to put a stop to being victimized, manipulated or dictated to. The universe isn't out to get you: you aren't powerless.

Stop pretending you're an ostrich with your head in the sand: no more hiding from your problems. Allow yourself to be seen and heard. Sardonyx encourages you to stand up and be unapologetic about what you believe in because your voice counts. It's time to start asserting yourself as a leader. When you step into your power, you no longer need external validation and can start living your purpose.

Your physiology affects your psychology and vice versa; your body language influences how others react to you. Strike a power-pose and stand like your ultimate superhero would. Take up as much space as you need. Doing so is proven to make you feel more confident and will have a positive effect on how people respond to you. This energy is supercharged: it will manifest new opportunities and friendships, and improve close relationships.

*Be your own superhero*

| | |
|---|---|
| **PHYSICAL HEALING:** | Believed to enhance physical strength, stamina and muscle tone when exercising; removes blockages and toxins, fortifies the blood and remedies sexual dysfunction |
| **CHAKRA:** | Base |
| **SOURCE:** | Brazil, Germany, India, Russia, Uruguay and USA |

# SELENITE

## Purifying, harmonizing, calming, nurturing

Selenite's name comes from the Greek word *selene*, meaning 'moon'. Maybe it's because it looks as if it's made of frozen moonbeams. Its radiant energy is perfect for giving your vibes a spring clean. Selenite is an everyday crystal that you can use morning, noon and night. One of its superpowers is the ability to dissolve 'blocks': if you're feeling stuck, meditate with Selenite in the morning so that you start the day feeling bright-eyed and bushy-tailed.

If you have a large wand-like piece of Selenite you can use it as a lightsaber for a mid-afternoon pick-me-up: wave it around your body and imagine it hoovering up any unwanted energy that might be making you feel foggy. You could also use it to energetically cleanse your workspace, laptop, phone or home of any discordant energy in the same way. Do this if you've been experiencing a creative block, you've received a rude email or you're getting frustrated with your job/life/relationship. Cleanse those vibes so that you can start flowing again. Keep a piece of Selenite in your bedroom or living room to help you decompress from the day's events and chill without any distractions. Sleeping with Selenite can support a restful night so you wake up feeling fresh and energized.

Hanging out with Selenite may help you tune into your intuition and guide you to go deeper with your meditations. It's all about feeling calmer and more balanced so that you can access your channels of inspiration. Keep Selenite with you if you want to connect with your spirit guides. Use the internet to find a guided meditation that's designed to connect you with them; set up your crystal altar (see page 72), light some candles and incense, make sure you won't be disturbed and place your Selenite either above your head to open your crown chakra or on your forehead to activate your third eye (you'll need to be lying down to keep it in place), follow the meditation and call in your spiritual support team. Make sure you record your experience afterwards.

*Being quiet and still allows you to connect to higher guidance*

| | |
|---|---|
| **PHYSICAL HEALING:** | **Believed to calm hyperactivity and ADHD, balance hormones, enhance fertility and remedy PMS, period and menopausal symptoms** |
| **CHAKRA:** | **Crown, third eye and sacral** |
| **SOURCE:** | **Australia, Greece, Mexico and USA** |

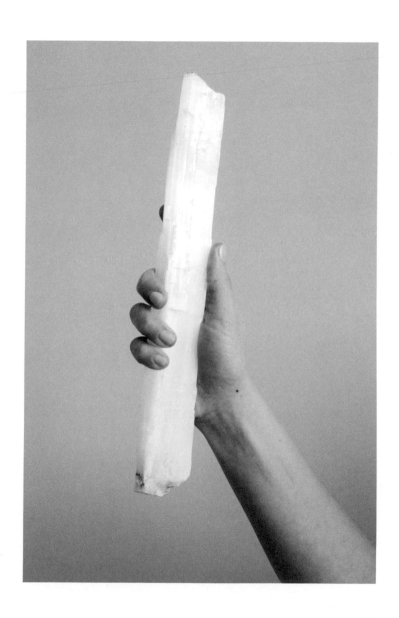

SELENITE

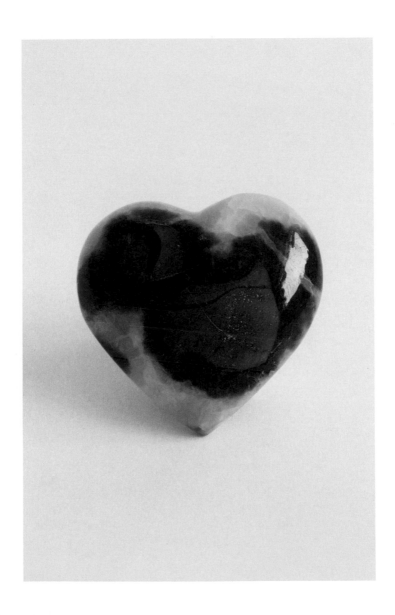

# SEPTARIAN (DRAGON STONE)

## Protective, grounding, calming, confidence, happy, adventure

Septarian is a fusion of yellow Calcite, Aragonite and limestone. It's a cheerful collaboration of energies that can make you feel grounded and uplifted.

This is a happy-go-lucky stone that brings your attention to the power of the here and now to change things and make a difference. Septarian is all about making your lofty dreams reality. Yes, they may seem unachievable and overwhelming now but break it all down into bite-sized tasks. Get a pen and paper, write down what you can do today, tomorrow, next week and the month after to start putting the wheels in motion. Create a Pinterest board to collect your ideas, look out for courses that will give you the tools to succeed, buy the domain so that you've got somewhere for your website, research suppliers and reach out to people who inspire you to see if they can advise you. Be innovative with the resources you have available to you now, instead of waiting for the right time to start. Today's the day.

Septarian can awaken your sense of adventure and encourage you to be open to where the journey will take you. It's about making new friends and getting out into nature. It reminds you to be more mindful in your interactions, slowing down to be grateful for what you have and to savour the beauty within each and every moment. See also Aragonite (page 128).

*You already have everything that you need to succeed*

| PHYSICAL HEALING: | Believed to promote self-healing, strengthen teeth and bones, and accelerate the repair of broken bones |
| --- | --- |
| CHAKRA: | Solar plexus and base |
| SOURCE: | Australia, Canada, England, Madagascar, New Zealand and USA |

# SHATTUCKITE

## Channelling, shamanic, intuition, divination, protection

Shattuckite has a shamanic energy and activates your third eye, offering protection as you connect to altered states of consciousness via meditation and journeying. This stone is stabilizing and grounding, supporting you while you're tuning into spiritual energies. It enhances intuitive abilities and can help if you're studying esoteric practices, such as tarot, astrology, runes and other forms of divination. If you're doing psychic readings, healing treatments or working with the tarot, Shattuckite will help you zone out from any distractions so that you're a clear channel to tune into other energies. It will help you to interpret your visions and the information you download from Spirit.

You don't need a crystal ball or to be in meditation to receive messages from the universe, though: every day can be a vision quest when you observe synchronicities and omens around you, including animals that cross your path and how often you see angel numbers (which are repeated numbers, like 111, 222, 333). Sometimes the answers can come to you in the shower. Everything has a meaning when you take time to acknowledge the signs and what they signify to you.

*Delve into your psychic skills and see where they lead you*

| | |
|---|---|
| **PHYSICAL HEALING:** | **Believed to assist with infections and reduce inflammation in the nose, ears, mouth and throat** |
| **CHAKRA:** | **Third eye, throat and heart** |
| **SOURCE:** | **Argentina, Austria, Germany, Greece, Namibia, Norway, South Africa, UK and USA** |

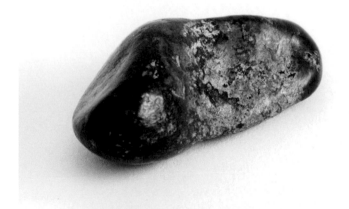

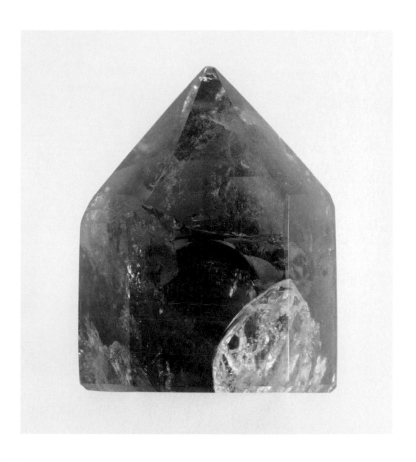

PHYSICAL
HEALING:
Said to relieve chronic pain, enhance well-being,
reduce inflammation, alleviate the effects of radiation
therapies and exposure to electromagnetic pollution

CHAKRA: Crown and base

SOURCE: Australia, Brazil, Madagascar, Switzerland and USA

# SMOKY QUARTZ

## Confidence, self-acceptance, empowerment, protection, grounding

Smoky Quartz is a protective, grounding and stabilizing crystal. It is the kind of friend who tells you exactly how it is, instead of what you want to hear, the truth you knew deep down anyway. It will put you back into the driver's seat of your own life so that you can feel you've got a say in where you're heading.

If you're a procrastinator and *mañana* (meaning 'morning' or 'tomorrow' in Spanish) is your mantra, Smoky Quartz can open your eyes to the power of now. Hint: stop waiting for tomorrow. You don't need to change: it's time to start leaning into everything that's perfect right here, right now. This is your call to start shining your light with a whole lotta attitude. You've got the power!

Smoky Quartz will help you realize that challenges are transformative opportunities: the universe isn't against you, it's just nudging you to start doing things differently. Take some time to meditate, pull a tarot/oracle card, do something that connects with your highest self or talk things out with your truth-telling bestie. When you wake up to see the bigger picture, everything expands.

The impossible becomes possible when you tune in and commit to taking action towards what you want. This doesn't mean you need to make a grand leap by quitting your job or moving to the other side of the world: you can break your goals into small, realistic steps that feel right for you. Incremental changes that create grounded transformation.

I'd read that Smoky Quartz has the power to reduce pain. I'll admit that I was totally sceptical until I'd meditated with it when I had a sore throat and it actually took the pain away – the effect lasted more than twelve hours. I've since led a workshop focused on Smoky Quartz and one of my friends, who suffers from a chronic condition, reported that her pain had been radically reduced after the workshop. I'm not a medical professional and I'm definitely not recommending that you come off your medication in the hope of Smoky Quartz saving the day: I would suggest you incorporate this crystal into your routine for some extra support. You could meditate (see page 64) with Smoky Quartz or create a layout (page 90) and visualize it easing any pain or discomfort; you could create a crystal elixir (page 96) or soak in a nice warm bath infused with Smoky Quartz and salt minerals to soothe your body.

Use Smoky Quartz's detoxing effect to purify any electromagnetic stress. Keep it by your phone, laptop or electrical equipment to absorb and protect you from unwanted radiation.

*Transformation comes when you believe in yourself and dare to shine*

# SODALITE

## Problem-solving, insight, honesty

Sodalite is believed to stimulate your intellect and empathy. Its calming energy will help you concentrate and retain new information, making it a useful crystal for students, teachers, writers, therapists and researchers. It can quieten your mind and clear distractions so you're able to focus on tasks that may at first seem overwhelming.

Meditating with Sodalite may help you identify your subconscious patterns and motives so you have more clarity. It can demystify whatever is stopping you moving forward, and is an ally in problem-solving.

Use Sodalite to expand your awareness of other people's needs and to communicate with them in an honest, compassionate way.

This stone activates the throat chakra and will support you in expressing yourself confidently, so it's ideal for public speaking, acting and remembering lines.

*The answers will come to you when you quiet your mind and listen*

PHYSICAL HEALING: **Thought to alleviate symptoms of menopause and reduce high blood pressure**

CHAKRA: **Throat and heart**

SOURCE: **Bahia, Brazil, Canada, India, Namibia and USA**

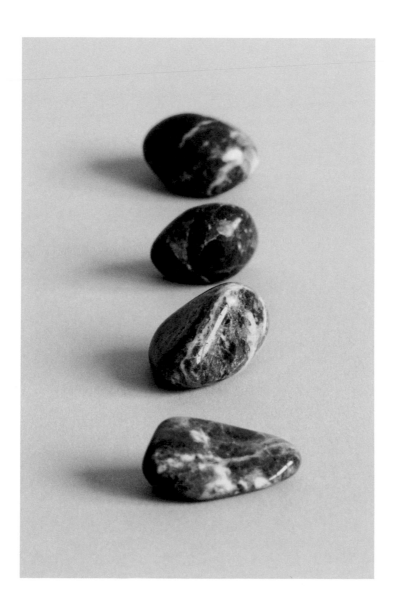

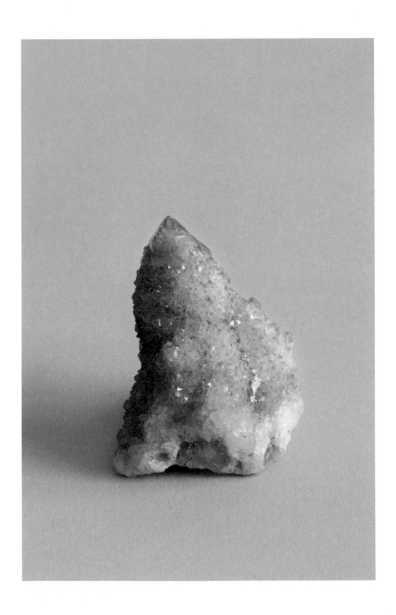

# SPIRIT QUARTZ
# (CACTUS QUARTZ)

## Spiritual connection, intuition, synchronicity, joy

Spirit Quartz has tiny shimmering points that reflect harmonizing energy in every direction. Its energy is gentle and uplifting, and can be used to press reset when you're feeling stressed or overwhelmed. Spirit Quartz is a crystal that can put you back in the flow-lane with the universe after you've been sidetracked by dramas and disasters. It will help you dust yourself off so that you feel ready to rejoin the party.

Remember to infuse some fun into whatever you're doing and to laugh. Laugh as much as you can – it's one of the best medicines and it's *free*, of course. It can flip your mood in an instant. Life doesn't have to be so serious. Spirit Quartz will spring clean your energy and declutter any negative attachments so you feel aligned with the Now and are wide-eyed to synchronicities.

It's time to start measuring your success by how much fun you're having. You don't have to conform to society's standards of the 'perfect' life. Set your spirit free and be the master of your own destiny: you don't need anyone's permission to be yourself. Embrace the fact that your life doesn't have to look like anyone else's. Spirit Quartz invites you to let go of any judgement or comparison so you can be more compassionate to others and yourself. It brings people together: collaboration instead of competition.

This crystal has the power to activate your third eye and open your crown chakra to switch on your intuition, connecting you to cosmic energies. Meditate with this crystal and invite your spirit guides to come and say hello. Use the internet to find a guided meditation that's designed to connect you with your spirit guides: set up your crystal altar (see page 72), light some candles and incense, make sure you won't be disturbed and place your Spirit Quartz either above your head to open your crown chakra or on your forehead to activate your third eye (you'll need to be lying down to keep it in place), follow the meditation and call in your spiritual support team. Make sure you record your experience afterwards.

*Your vibe attracts your tribe*

| | |
|---|---|
| **PHYSICAL HEALING:** | **Promotes general well-being** |
| **CHAKRA:** | **Crown, third eye and solar plexus** |
| **SOURCE:** | **South Africa** |

# SUNSTONE

## Energizing, action, confidence, socializing

Yearning for brighter days, when life's simple and your hardest decision is which cocktail to sip? If you can't escape into the sun, get some Sunstone into your life. Imagine sunshine breaking through the clouds on a rainy day and warming your skin: that's how this portable sunbeam will make you feel. It's your crystal vitamin D to give you a boost when it's grey outside – or maybe when life's been shades of grey, regardless of the weather forecast.

Sunstone is energizing and can supercharge your vibes to bring back your *joie de vivre*. It's known to activate your solar plexus and sacral chakras, making you feel more confident and sociable. Has your social calendar been a little flat lately? Hop into the group chat with your favourite friends and hook up for a night out for some much-needed fun and laughter.

You may be drawn to Sunstone if you're being called to step into your power: it's time to let your confidence shine through so that people can see what you're really capable of. Stop putting yourself in the shade. This could mean proposing a new project to your team, going for a promotion or making the moves to start your own side hustle.

Sunstone invites abundance into your life, which can come in many forms and in unexpected ways. It may make you feel more generous and want to share with others.

This stone's radiant energy might even inspire you to take a break and book a trip somewhere the sun is guaranteed to be shining. Everything's better when the sun's out, and with this stone you can keep that energy with you, even when you're indoors at a desk.

*Take action and step into your power*

| | |
|---|---|
| **PHYSICAL HEALING:** | **Believed to improve digestion and increase metabolism, remedy stomach ailments, balance hormones and support reproductive health** |
| **CHAKRA:** | **Solar plexus and sacral** |
| **SOURCE:** | **Canada, India, Norway, Russia and USA** |

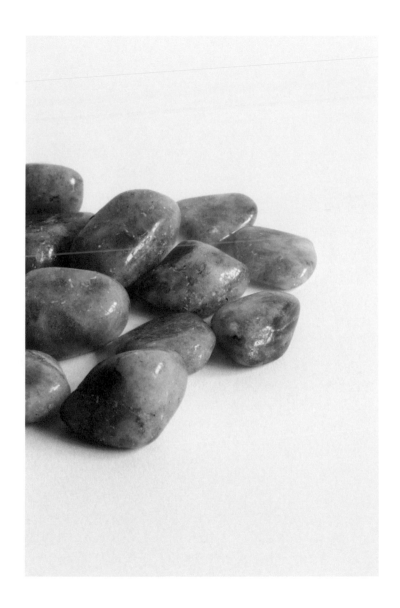

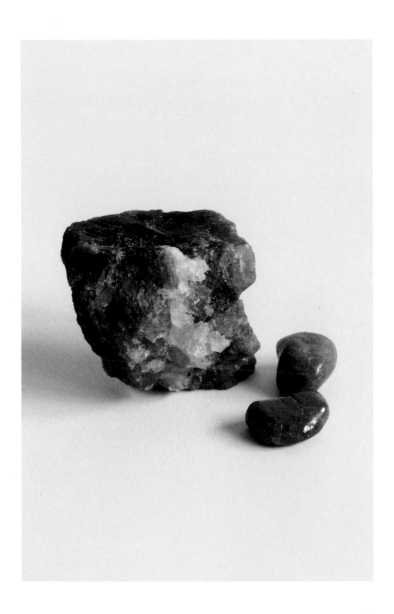

# TANZANITE

## Intuition, manifestation, uplifting, self-expression, adventure

Tanzanite is a high-vibration crystal that's spiritually activating. It can open your heart, crown and third eye chakras so you can attune to cosmic awareness. It's also said to clear your throat chakra to help you communicate your truth. After hanging out with Tanzanite, you'll feel like a butterfly stepping out from your cocoon. It's all about embracing everything that's unique about you instead of trying to conform to something that doesn't fit you any more.

This crystal will remind you that anything's possible: it's up to you to dream it and make it happen. When you allow yourself to go with the flow without the need for something to be perfect, inspiration and magic know exactly where to find you.

Explore your spiritual side: learn to meditate, go to a retreat somewhere like Bali, practise yoga, consult your tarot cards, have a Reiki treatment, experience a sound bath. Take some time out from your usual routine so that you can start tapping into cosmic energy. Take Tanzanite along for the ride: it may help you manifest all kinds of wonderful things and situations.

*Say yes to adventure!*

| | |
|---|---|
| **PHYSICAL HEALING:** | **Believed to detoxify, boost the immune system, increase cellular regeneration of hair, skin and nails, and alleviate adrenal fatigue** |
| **CHAKRA:** | **Crown, third eye, throat and heart** |
| **SOURCE:** | **Africa** |

# TIGER'S EYE

## Confidence, empowerment, boundaries

Tiger's Eye is like the life coach of the crystal realm because it's a confidence-boosting crystal that will support you in stepping out of your comfort zone and opening you up to life-changing experiences. It's like an accountability buddy that can hold you to doing the things you say you will and give you the courage to say yes to new opportunities, instead of shying away and hiding. This is definitely one to sleep with under your pillow the night before a job interview or if you're asking for a promotion.

As you feel more empowered, you'll start being more decisive and learn to trust your judgement, discerning what's right for you. There's no room left for anxiety. It's time to take control of your life. Each time you say yes to what *you* want, you'll strengthen your confidence muscle.

This stone loves to help you focus on your goals and say no to things that drain your energy – it's an ideal stone for people-pleasers. Tiger's Eye may support you in resisting peer pressure, and help you say no to doing things that waste your time or that you don't want to do. If you don't want to go for after-work drinks with your colleagues because you'd rather go home to your cat, do that. Instead of feeling guilty, start leaning into being okay with 'selfishness'. Team Tiger's Eye with Amethyst (see page 117) for more willpower to help overcome addictions and support positive new habits.

Tiger's Eye is also a grounding stone that will give you strength if you're feeling victimized or bullied. Keep this stone with you when you need to protest about something you believe in and speak up against any injustices.

*Turn down the volume of your fears so that you can start moving forward*

| PHYSICAL HEALING: | Said to stimulate and strengthen the body, balance hormones and promote a sense of vigour |
|---|---|
| CHAKRA: | Solar plexus, sacral and base |
| SOURCE: | Australia, India, Myanmar, South Africa and USA |

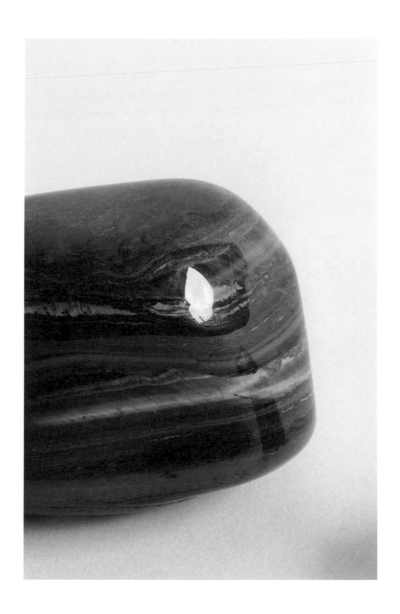

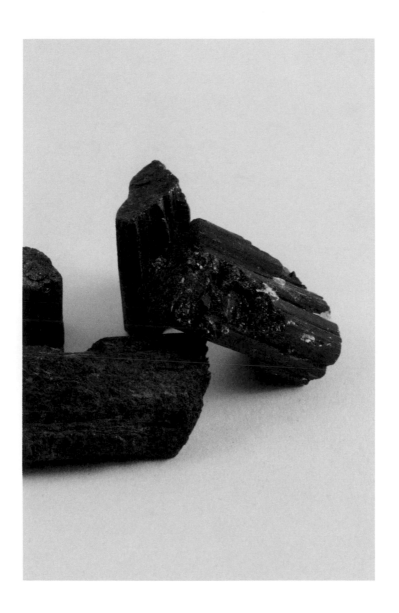

# TOURMALINE – BLACK

## Grounding, protection, anxiety, panic attacks, confidence, support

Hanging out with Black Tourmaline is like getting a huge bear hug from the universe that makes you feel grounded and protected. This stone can encourage you to integrate the shadow aspects of yourself. Have some nasty thoughts been running your show? They might be thoughts of comparison, jealousy, low self-worth, fear of failure, financial insecurity and anxiety (which most of us have at some point). What you don't own owns you, so use Black Tourmaline to practise self-acceptance and compassion. Tune into what these triggers are showing you because these situations are just lessons waiting to be understood. By honouring the light *and* the dark within, you'll stop feeling fragmented and learn how to truly love yourself.

Black Tourmaline wants you to start putting yourself first, instead of worrying about what other people think. Always bending to other people's demands drains your energy and is a huge anxiety trigger: it makes you feel invisible and helpless. It's safe to say no, especially if it means that you're saying yes to something that supports you.

You've got to put on your own life jacket before you can rescue anyone else.

*Take back control of your life – stand up for yourself*

| | |
|---|---|
| **PHYSICAL HEALING:** | Said to detoxify pollutants that could cause illness and disease; has a pain-relieving benefit |
| **CHAKRA:** | Base |
| **SOURCE:** | Africa, Brazil, Nepal and USA |

# TURQUOISE

## Hope, protection, healing, tribe, union

The stunning blue and green hues of turquoise are so soothing and tranquil. You're momentarily a castaway swimming in crystal-clear waters without a care in the world when this stone catches your eye. It has the power to slow everything down and tune out any distractions, reconnecting you with the here and now. It's mesmerizing because we don't get this feeling often enough.

It is said that turquoise formed when Native Americans danced to celebrate the arrival of long-awaited rain: their tears of happiness mixed with the rain, which was absorbed by the earth to create Fallen Sky Stone, or Turquoise. Apaches associated it with rain at the end of the rainbow. Indigenous tribes revered Turquoise as sacred, the connection between heaven and earth. They'd wear it as a talisman for protection, to make them invisible as hunters and stronger warriors. It was also used for communicating with spirits, healing and good fortune.

Turquoise connects us with spiritual wisdom. It reminds us to walk our path as brothers and sisters to each other, with a side order of compassion and forgiveness. We need to wake up to our lifestyle choices and how they impact on Mother Earth. Turquoise reminds us of the beauty of our planet and that we need to enforce more acts of preservation to keep it safe for all of the living creatures we share it with.

Work with Turquoise to tune into your inner shaman: it will guide you into deep meditations so that you can connect with ancestors, spirit guides and the elements for guidance and healing.

*Share your heart with the earth*

| PHYSICAL HEALING: | Said to boost the immune system and nutrient absorption; uplifting and supportive energy for sufferers of depression, anxiety and panic attacks |
| --- | --- |
| CHAKRA: | Throat and heart |
| SOURCE: | Chile, China, Iran, Mexico, Tibet and USA |

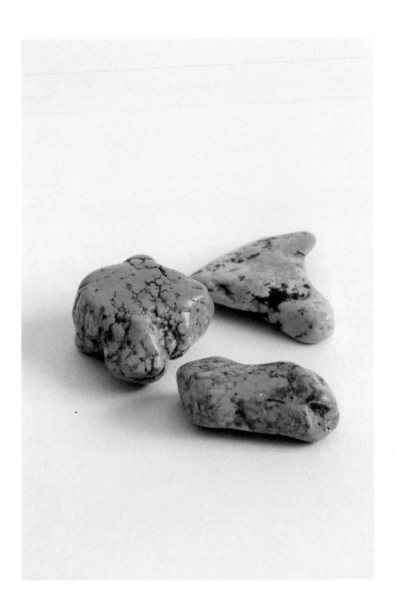

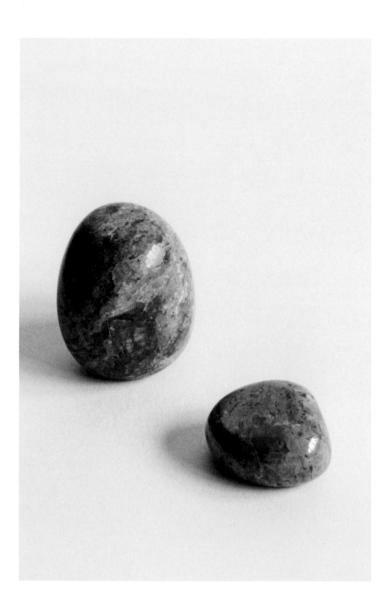

# UNAKITE

## Balance, love, harmony, communication, compassion

Unakite is a combination of Red Jasper, Epidote and, occasionally, Quartz. It's a stone that unites the heart and mind, bringing balance and harmony to your relationships.

Unakite's energy is slow and steady, teaching patience and surrender. It makes space for your inner child, the parts of you that may be feeling neglected and wanting attention. Is a situation coming up in your life when you want to have everything your way? When you're working with Unakite, instead of holding grudges or questioning what the future has in store, focus on what's true in the moment. You don't need to do things the hard way. It can guide you to communicate your needs and feelings, to prevent potential tantrums and meltdowns. This is a great stone for little and big kids alike.

If you're a self-confessed control freak, work with Unakite to help you loosen your grip on your to-do list. It will encourage you to delegate and streamline so that you have more space to create with a clear mind. Let yourself be supported by this crystal (and the people around you).

*Live in the now and forgive yourself for any past mistakes*

| | |
|---|---|
| **PHYSICAL HEALING:** | **Believed to increase vitality, stimulate self-healing and cell regeneration; supports the heart, blood, immune system, fertility and health during pregnancy and labour** |
| **CHAKRA:** | **Heart, solar plexus and sacral** |
| **SOURCE:** | **Brazil, France, Germany, India, Russia and USA** |

# CHAPTER FOUR

# CRYSTAL COLOURS AND MEANINGS

If the crystal you're looking for doesn't appear in this guide, one of the easiest ways to interpret the medicine of your chosen stone is to study its colour. In the same way that hearing a song on the radio can evoke a memory or feeling, or a scent can spark nostalgia, colours have their own resonance.

Crystals absorb and reflect light energy. When rays of light pass through them, some of the wavelengths are filtered and absorbed; the rays that remain are what you see as the stone's colour. This colour is a facet of each crystal's personality. Soft- and pastel-coloured crystals will be more calming and nurturing, while bright, bold-coloured stones will be more dynamic and stimulating.

## CHECK MY GUIDE FOR WHAT YOU CAN EXPECT FROM EACH SHADE OF CRYSTAL AND HOW IT CAN HELP YOU:

### CLEAR/COLOURLESS

Promotes clarity, cleansing and new beginnings. This colour is healing, amplifies energy and supports innovation, well-being and spiritual development. Use it to work with spirit guides and angels.

### WHITE

Represents purity and nurturing – ideal for emotional healing, new beginnings, hope, soothing, balancing and supporting new mothers.

### BLACK

Use black stones for protection, to absorb and shield negative energy; grounding; transformation work with your shadow side, and to support you through trauma, grief and pain.

### GREY

Supports neutrality, balance, adaptability, justice, compromise and objectivity.

### RED

Supports action, commitment, passion, sexuality, fertility and courage, as well as stability, grounding, endurance and leadership.

### ORANGE

Helps with creativity, fertility, joy, self-expression, sexuality, confidence, personal development and is energizing.

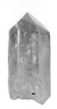

### YELLOW

Promotes happiness, joy, optimism and abundance, as well as helping with confidence, gratitude, energy, setting health boundaries, improving memory and manifestation.

### GREEN

Helps with balance, connecting to nature, healing, grounding and creating a sense of well-being, love, prosperity, abundance; opens you up to new ventures.

### PINK

Use to create and attract love, kindness, appreciation, compassion and balance; opens your heart to resolve disagreements and promotes forgiveness, self-acceptance and appreciation.

### BLUE

Enhances communication, loyalty, leadership, expression and compassion; soothes, calms and also boosts mental clarity.

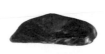

## PURPLE

Use to open up to your psychic senses, spiritual development and intuition; calms, helps in overcoming addictions and obsessive thinking; soothes anxiety and headaches.

## BROWN

Grounding and practical, supporting humanitarian endeavours; helps in slowing things down.

## GOLD

Attracts abundance and prosperity in all forms; helps energize and increases confidence and new opportunities.

## SILVER

Soothes, balances and cleanses; boosts intuition and supports all things feminine and linked to lunar cycles.

## IRIDESCENT

Activates all of your chakras, and helps with creativity, inspiration, self-expression and confidence.

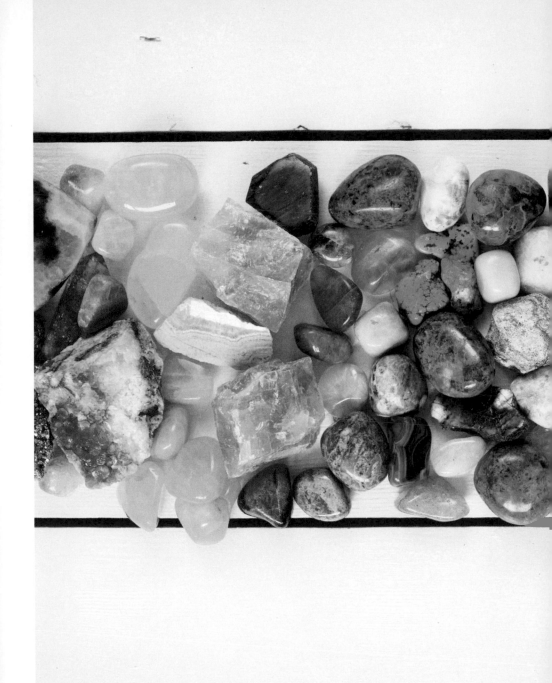

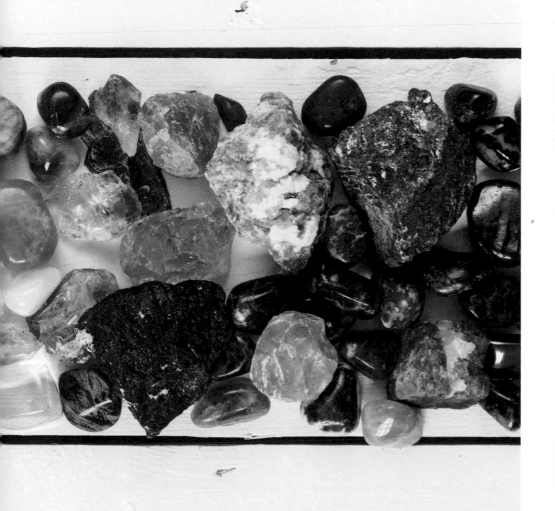

# CHAPTER FIVE

# CONCLUSION

Crystals can be life-changing, but you'll be waiting for ever if you're hoping for your life to be radically transformed by carrying a hunk of Rose Quartz around in your handbag. We aren't here to wish on crystals. We're here to be crystal activists, collaborating with crystal-kind to bring all kinds of wonder to life.

A crystal is just the tip of an iceberg. What lies beneath it are your motives, hopes, dreams, desires, aspirations and challenges. Crystals will catch your attention because they're full of juicy promises and you want to get in on the good vibes, especially when it seems as if the universe is bestowing blessings on everyone but you.

I'll be the first to admit that crystals are addictive: it's so tempting to keep adding to your collection until you can't put a mug of tea on your bedside table.

Crystals are like cosmic life coaches; they all have their own opinion about how you can empower yourself and resolve any perpetuating challenges. Imagine a squad of crystals, all with useful advice but they're all coming from different perspectives. We've all done it: asked everyone's advice about a situation hoping to get the answer we want to hear rather than acknowledging the truth we know deep down. It's common to approach crystals in the same way: 'If I buy these crystals then hopefully my problems will disappear.' That's bypassing responsibility for your life and not fully trusting your intuition. It leads to an expanding crystal collection, alongside a crystal graveyard (or the dusty trinket bowl where crystals go to be forgotten) with hopes that the latest rock star you've bought is the missing piece of the puzzle. Alas, nothing changes. Maybe this crystal healing thing is a scam after all.

Let's say you're unhappy at work: this job was a stopgap that's turned into three years of your life, your anxiety is at its peak and you don't know what to do next. Citrine might say, 'Quit people-pleasing and start looking for a new job'; Celestite might say, 'Chill out and ask for help'; and Black Tourmaline might say, 'Stop judging yourself and bring some boundaries in so that work isn't overflowing into your personal time.'

It's all great advice but it's like trying to cook three different recipes in a single oven. You can't fit it all in. Overwhelming, huh? I'm here to tell you that you don't need them all. More crystals does not equal a fast-pass to enlightenment and all of your dreams coming true. The biggest lesson I've learnt about crystals is that you only really need one (or a few) at a time. Get to know one, follow its lead and you'll be doing your best impression of Gollum before you know it. Everything's easier when you take it one step/crystal at a time.

Consider where your motive is coming from. Your heart or your ego? Instead of choosing a crystal to 'fix' or change something, what about choosing a crystal that brings to life the parts of your personality that you've always been too shy to reveal or to embrace the parts of yourself that you don't like? Crystal healing is all about getting to know the real you.

My favourite thing about crystals is the way they activate our intuition. Last summer, I led a series of workshops on an island in Croatia. Nestled in the Adriatic Sea, this place is a hidden gem (literally); it has exposed Calcite formations that run through it. It isn't often that we get to be up close and personal with crystals in their native environment because they're usually already mined and shop-ready when we find them. On the night of the full moon, I led a guided meditation (a.k.a. a journey) on the beach. As part of that journey I asked the group to visualize a crystal at the centre of the earth waiting for them. It could be any size, shape or colour. I invited them to witness what came to their thoughts in those moments. Later some meditators came up to me, curious about the crystals they'd seen in their visions.

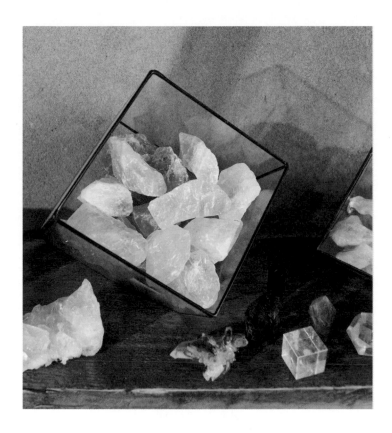

One of the girls recalled that she'd seen a purple clustered crystal and we agreed that it might have been Amethyst. I told her that Amethyst loves to support over-thinkers and she laughed. 'I'm definitely an over-thinker!' They were surprised that I could tell so much about them from what they'd experienced in the meditation. All I was doing was translating the crystals as I know them to serve as prompts in unravelling the visions. Intuitively, they'd all connected with a crystal that wanted to support them, without any experience with crystals or the actual crystals close to hand. Like a trippy Hall of Mirrors, but instead of showing bodies distorted into different shapes and sizes, they were reflected as a crystal.

# 'My favourite thing about crystals is the way they activate our intuition'

The truth is: you always know what you need, even if it isn't obvious. You just need to be still enough to notice.

Choose your crystals based on the things that make your heart go boom-boom.

Certain crystals will feel familiar because you'll be reminded of times when they had your back. That's how I remember crystals: like Moonstone (see page 202) when my life felt like an emotional rollercoaster and I was burning the candle at both ends; Kunzite (page 185) when I could sense that things weren't going to work out with a guy I was seeing, and then when I got together with my boyfriend (now) and all of my insecurities came bubbling to the surface – he actually chose a Kunzite pendant for me at a crystal fair without knowing what it was for! Labradorite (page 189) has helped when I've been sinking in a quicksand pit of comparison and imposter syndrome. These crystals inspired me to do something about whatever was wrong and helped me to stay woke, instead of falling back into old habits. Moonstone led me to counselling and exploring other forms of personal development so that I can recognize my triggers and patterns; Kunzite led me to a book called *Spirit Junkie* by Gabrielle Bernstein that changed my relationship, enabled us still to be together four years later; and Labradorite encouraged me to take a social media detox so that I could get back in my own lane and focus on writing this book that you're reading.

Crystals have also been brought to life for me by the people I've given them to and how their situation played out after they'd received them; by my clients and their experiences in session; and by the stories that people share in the crystal workshops I lead, when they're in awe of how much they've understood about their situation just from meditating with a crystal.

# 'You always know what you need, even if it isn't obvious. You just need to be still enough to notice'

When you choose a crystal, you're giving yourself permission to want that particular thing in your life. The crystals will hold space for you to expand your belief system around what you're entitled to experience, like being in a relationship where you can both be 100 per cent yourselves, without judgement or compromise, you fancy the pants off each other and you share a vision for the future; a career that flexes all of your superpowers and your work–life balance is on point; travelling the world and learning from other cultures; being part of a community; finding inner peace and fulfilment; making a positive difference. All crystals want you to do is commit to yourself. Because that's where real change comes from, not just for us as individuals but for the whole planet.

Don't rely entirely on this book to teach you everything you need to know about crystals. Within these pages, some, all or nothing of what I share with you will resonate. My word is not gospel. In the words of Albert Einstein, 'The only source of knowledge is experience.' We're all here to have our own experience. You don't need to study all of the books and online resources to understand what a crystal is saying: you need to take them off the shelf and get to know the ones you've got. They've come into your life for a reason.

I'd love it if you referred back to this book until it's dog-eared because you've used the information, the meditations, rituals and practices to follow your own journey, but it wouldn't be complete without a sidekick: your journal, full of your crystal musings, visions and 'aha' moments. In the same way that a dream can feel vivid when you first wake up and fades as soon as you dive into your day, it's easy to forget what you've experienced. Write it all down. Your notes will act as seeds that allow the crystals' messages to blossom. Think of it as notes to your future self that will remind you, again and again, your intuition knows best.

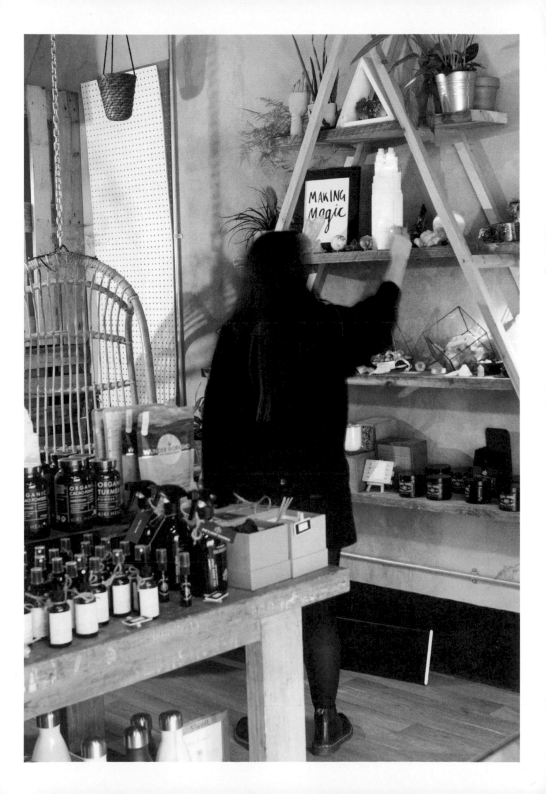

# CRYSTAL INDEX

# ACKNOWLEDGEMENTS

To Fang, for literally building a house around me while I typed away on my laptop. I'm so grateful that the crystal 'love spell' brought you into my life. Thank you for grounding me while giving me the freedom to spread my wings. I love you.

To my mum, for forever giving me space to be myself and supporting me in every way you could. To Sarah, for always being there to guide me.

There are so many incredible people who have supported me along this wild ride. Thank you for reminding me that none of us have it all figured out but at least we've got each other. You mean the world to me and you know who you are.

To all of my teachers, thank you for inspiring me, sharing your wisdom, and giving me the tools to embrace life to the fullest. You have helped me to become the person that I am today.

White Star, I'm infinitely grateful to you for teaching me how to speak to the spirits and crystals.

Elizabeth McKenzie and Laura Jane Williams – thank you for being my writing guides and teaching me that a shitty first draft is key in letting the story unfold.

Valeria Huerta, my agent, you brought this book to life. Thank you for seeing something in me that I hadn't thought possible and for your determination and support throughout the whole process. Thank you to Emily Robertson, my editor at Penguin Life. You shared my vision from the start – I knew you were the one! To her assistant, Rosanna, and to the rest of the incredible team at Penguin Random House who've been in involved in the creation of *The Crystal Code*; I haven't even met you all but I'm so grateful for your talents.

Thank you Kristina Sälgvik, for capturing the beauty of these crystals with your brilliant photography skills.

Cheryl Eltringham and Jill Urwin of She's Lost Control – I'm beyond grateful for all of the magic that we've been able to create together over the last three years! Thank you for allowing us to use some of your treasures for the photoshoot and to take some pictures at She's Lost Control HQ. **@SLC_London www.sheslostcontrol.co.uk**

Buddha on a Bicycle for lending us your most prized crystals to be featured in the book – thank you. **@BuddhaonBicycle www.buddhaonabicycle.com**

Ruby Warrington and The Numinous for inviting me to share my story and giving me the opportunity to write about mystical topics on the site. Your portal allows us to see the medicine in our own stories.

Finally, I want to send love beams of gratitude to all of those who've attended my workshops, my clients, my instagram tribe and those that hold this book in their hands. Thank you for sharing this space with me while we unlock our superpowers with crystals by our side!!

# ABOUT
# THE AUTHOR

Tamara Driessen is a crystal healer, shamanic practitioner, reiki master and tarot advisor. She trained with a shaman in Bali and now runs regular moon ceremonies and crystal healing workshops in the UK and beyond. She is a resident teacher at the modern lifestyle and mindfulness curator, She's Lost Control, a contributor to The Numinous and a founding member of the Obonjan wellness festival. She has collaborated with brands such as Topshop and Vice and leads bespoke intuitive/mystical guidance and healing sessions with a wide range of clients.

🐦 @__wolfsister

ⓕ @wolfsisterhealing

📷 __wolfsister

www.wolfsister.com